VEGAN SLOW COOKER RECIPES

Vegan Quick and Easy Gluten Free Low Cholesterol Whole Foods Recipes

(Easy High Protein Tasty Recipes for Fast Weight Loss)

Theresa Veliz

Published by Sharon Lohan

© Theresa Veliz

All Rights Reserved

Vegan Slow Cooker Recipes: Vegan Quick and Easy Gluten Free Low Cholesterol Whole Foods Recipes (Easy High Protein Tasty Recipes for Fast Weight Loss)

ISBN 978-1-990334-35-1

All rights reserved. No part of this guide may be reproduced in any form without permission in writing from the publisher except in the case of brief quotations embodied in critical articles or reviews.

Legal & Disclaimer

The information contained in this book is not designed to replace or take the place of any form of medicine or professional medical advice. The information in this book has been provided for educational and entertainment purposes only.

The information contained in this book has been compiled from sources deemed reliable, and it is accurate to the best of the Author's knowledge; however, the Author cannot guarantee its accuracy and validity and cannot be held liable for any errors or omissions. Changes are periodically made to this book. You must consult your doctor or get professional medical advice before using any of the suggested remedies, techniques, or information in this book.

Table of contents

Part 1 1
Introduction 2
"Where Do You Get Your Protein?" 2
"Can You Eat This?" 5
"Is This Really Vegan?" 6
"Is Being Vegan Expensive?" 8
"Is Being Vegan A Lot Of Work?" 10
Slow Cooker Tips 11
Breakfast 13
Vegan Omelet 13
Breakfast Casserole 14
Stuffed Apples 15
Coffee Cake 17
Crockpot Oatmeal 19
Breakfast Brownies 20
Beverages 22
Gingerbread Latte 22
Peppermint Hot Chocolate 23
Hot Buttered Rum 25
Horchata Latte 26
Soups 28
Ginger Carrot Soup 28

Split Pea Soup	29
Corn Chowder	30
Loaded Baked Potato Soup	32
Homey Tomato Soup	34
Turmeric Apple Soup	35
Main Courses	37
Butternut Squash Alfredo	37
Coconut Curry	38
Protein-Packed Chili	40
Masala Lentils	42
Tomato Basil Risotto	43
Stuffed Acorn Squash	45
Vegan Lo-Mein	46
Mushroom Bourguignon	48
Vegan Stroganoff	50
Truffle Oil Mac & Cheese	51
Veggie Fajitas	53
Hearty Meatloaf	54
Cottage Pie	55
Garlic Spaghetti Squash	57
Loaded Potatoes	58
Vegan Lasagna	60
Butternut Dahl	61
White Bean Orzo	62

"Butter" Chickpeas 63

Sides 65

Glazed Brussels Sprouts 65

Baked Sweet Potatoes 67

Jamaican Rice And Beans 68

Maple Glazed Carrots 69

Stuffed Peppers 70

Buttery Mushroom Rice 71

Snack Mix 72

Southern Style Green Beans 74

Cajun Potatoes 75

Desserts 77

Apple Nachos 77

Chai Tea Pie 78

Hot Fudge Cake 80

Pumpkin Butter 81

Rosewater Yogurt 82

Poached Pears 84

Part 2 86

Introduction 87

The Benefits Of Using A Slow Cooker 89

Breakfast Recipes 91

Peach Granola Crumble 91

Healthy Breakfast Casserole 92

- Overnight Millet And Oats 93
- Chia Seed Energy Bar Recipe 95
- Vegan Pumpkin Spice Syrup 96
- Apple Crumble Breakfast Pudding 97
- Bean And Grain Recipes 99
- Baked Beans 99
- Vegan Chili 100
- Red Beans And Rice 101
- Three-Bean Vegan Chili 102
- Spicy Chipotle Black-Eyed Peas 104
- Wild Rice Medley 105
- Barley And Bean Tacos With Avocado Chipotle Cream 107
- Slow Cooker Almond Quinoa Curry 108
- Salads And Sides 111
- Slow-Cooked Mediterranean Zucchini Salad 111
- German Potato Salad 112
- Garlic Cauliflower Mashed Potatoes 113
- Farro Salad 114
- Tofu And Black Bean Taco Salad 116
- Thai Summer Squash Salad With Peanut- Sauce ... 117
- Stews And Chilis 119
- Vegan Four Bean Chili 119
- Mushroom Lentil Buckwheat Stew 121

Corn And Red Pepper Chowder	122
Lentil Chili	123
Black Bean And Quinoa Crock-Pot Stew	125
Lentil Cauliflower Stew	126
Root Vegetable And Tempeh Vegan Chili	128
Vegetable Recipes	130
Balsamic Pear, Mushroom, And Asparagus	130
Baked Sweet Potatoes	131
Enchilada Amaranth	132
Rosemary And Red Pepper Tofu	134
Quick And Easy Swiss Cauliflower	135
Tempeh With Apples, Sweet Potatoes, And Sauerkraut	136
Vegetable Red Curry	137
Mediterranean Stuffed Peppers	139
Summer Vegetable Succotash Recipe	140
Eggplant Lasagna	142
Soups And Bowls	143
Yellow Pea Soup	143
Lentil Tortilla Soup	144
Lemon Rosemary Lentil Soup	146
Lentil And Potato Soup	147
Butternut Squash And Parsnip Soup	149
Desserts	150

Caramel Poached Peaches 150
Lemon Blueberry Cake 151
Caramel Mocha Cheesecake 153
Triple Chocolate-Peanut Butter Pudding Cake 155
Apple Crisp 157
Turmeric Rice Pudding 158
Berry Cobbler 159
Mediterranean Stew 162
Fennel Soup With White Bean 163
"Turks" Eggplants 164
Exotic French Vegetable Soup 165
Three Been Chili 167
Crock Pot Mediterranean Stew 168
Couscous Mediterranean Stew 169
Mediterranean Vegetable Stew 170
Delightful Spinach Lentil Soup 171
More Delightful Spinach Brown Lentil Soup 172
Cannellini Bean Soup 173
Potato And Bell Pepper Vegetable Stew 174
Yummy Artichoke Pasta 175
The White Man Spread 176
Wintery Soup With Squash And Chickpea 177
The Amazing Minestrone Casserole 178
Method 178

Bulgur And Lentils 179
Greek-Style Veggies 179
Mr. Three Vegetarian Chili 180
The Brave Vegan Chili 181
Delicious Mediterranean Tomato Sauce 182
Spiced Apple Sauce... 183
Garbanzo Chili 184
The Spinach Lover's Marinara Sauce......................... 185
Delicious Root Vegetable Tagine................................. 185
Grandma's Vegetarian Chili 186
Black Beans And Rice 187

Part 1

Introduction

You've probably heard this question 101 times since you decided to make the ethical and sustainable choice to go vegan. Your answer is probably, "Umm… everything that doesn't come from animals?" People are usually flabbergasted by this, but the fact is that a lot of food is already vegan—and with a little creativity and the right ingredients, you can vegan-ify almost anything else.

People often think that being vegan is limiting or a diet, but that's just not the case. Most vegans love food; they just choose to make their ethics and values a priority when choosing what to eat.

If you're new to vegan cooking, you might have some questions, so before you jump into the delicious and easy recipes in this book, take some time to read the introduction for tips, tricks, and helpful information.

"Where Do You Get Your Protein?"

This is another annoying question that vegans get asked all of the time. People act like meat and dairy are the only sources of protein in the world!

The fact is that most people in developed countries actually get too much protein. If you're new to the vegan diet, you should spend some time counting protein and planning your meals to make sure you're getting enough, but rest assured that protein deficiency is relatively rare.

Amino acids are organic compounds responsible for a wide variety of processes in the body. When they bind together in long chains, they make proteins. While our bodies can produce many of their own amino acids, there are nine types which the human body cannot create on its own. This means that we rely on our food for these.

Something vegans should keep in mind is that not all sources of protein have all of the amino acids that you need. In fact, most don't. But no need to worry: As long as you are able to get all of these amino acids within one day, you should be fine.

Practically, that means that you can't rely on just one or two sources of protein a day. When you're eating vegan, a good rule of thumb is that each meal should have two kinds of protein. This may sound like trouble, but you'd be surprised how many foods contain protein. Once you get used to eating a vegan diet and creative cooking, getting enough protein is something you won't even think about.

Check with a nutritionist or online to find out how many grams of protein you should be eating in a day. To make things easier, each of the recipes in this cookbook details how many grams of protein are in a serving.

If you're sick of answering the protein question, check out these common vegan proteins, how to use them, and their nutritional benefits.

Black Beans

Did you know that the darker the color of a bean, the more antioxidants it has? Black beans are definitely a vegan staple. With 15 grams of protein per cooked cup, plus 15 grams of fiber, black beans are a great way to make a meal more filling. From Mexican food to brownies (that's right, brownies) this cookbook has plenty of recipes that integrate this filling bean.

Walnuts

Nuts and seeds are another source of protein for vegans. Rich in healthy fats and protein, this nut is a great snack or addition to a meal to help you feel full. Add crushed walnuts to desserts, pasta, or even pizza!

Quinoa

Quinoa might just be the king of vegan protein. Once eaten by Incan warriors, this seed (yes, quinoa is technically a seed, although it's served as a grain) serves up a complete amino acid group. That means that if you eat quinoa, you won't have to worry about combining proteins. Quinoa is great in salads, made into a veggie burger, or served with curry. You can even find pasta made out of quinoa at your local health food store.

Chickpeas

This versatile legume isn't just for hummus (although hummus is a delicious vegan staple you should master). Chickpeas have 14.5 grams of protein per cooked cup, plus 11 grams of fiber, manganese, and folate, a nutrient important for women. Chickpeas are great in curries, salads, stews, and so much more.

Oats

There's no vegan breakfast quite as delicious as oatmeal loaded with cinnamon and brown sugar, and that's hardly the only good thing about oats. Oats have been proven to help reduce cholesterol, so if you went vegan for your heart health (good move) you should add oats into your diet whenever you can. Gluten-free? No worries! You can easily find gluten-free oats and oat flour.

Tofu
Made from soy beans, tofu is a vegan classic, but most non-vegans turn their nose up at it. Why has tofu gotten such a bad reputation? Who knows, but with the recipes in this book, even your carnivorous friends will become tofu enthusiasts. With just 178 calories—but 12 grams of protein—per serving, no vegan diet is complete without tofu. Bread it, fry it, bake it, or blend it; the possibilities are endless, so get creative with this protein-packed treat.
Be sure to buy GMO-free tofu, as the health effects of consuming genetically modified soybeans are unclear.

Lentils
Lentils are a legume that appears across the world, from French cuisine to Indian food, and frequently in this cookbook. With 18 grams of protein per cooked cup, lentils are a perfect addition to stews, veggie burgers, salads, and meat replacements.

"Can You Eat This?"

The quick answer to this question is yes. As a vegan, you can technically eat anything; you just choose not to. Whether you chose to become vegan for health reasons, weight loss, the environment, your love of animals, or all of the above, don't let your lifestyle choice make you feel limited. With some practice and creativity, eating vegan can open new doors of culinary delights, rather than closing them.

"Is This Really Vegan?"

You may find yourself asking that when you're eating at a vegan restaurant. How can they make food so creamy, buttery, or cheesy without using dairy? The answer is vegan hacks. There are a few staples that every vegan should be familiar with. These staples help to emulate flavors not usually associated with a plant-based diet.

Once you've mastered these ingredients, you'll hear a chorus of "Is this really vegan?" at your next dinner party.

Cashews

No vegan pantry is complete without cashews. Soak these babies in water for a few hours, drain, and blend with herbs and spices to make creamy dipping sauces, or with sugar and cocoa powder for vegan ice cream. The high-protein possibilities are practically endless. Cashew "milk" shakes, anyone?

Nutritional Yeast

Nutritional yeast has a cheesy flavor, making it most vegans' first choice when it comes to cheese replacements. It's super-low in calories but high in protein, with just 40 calories and 3 grams of protein per tablespoon. Most vegans just can't live without nutritional yeast, and retailers know this; that's why it often comes fortified with vitamins that vegans tend to lack, like vitamin B_{12}. Why take a multivitamin if you can just eat creamy, delicious vegan queso every day?

Tahini

Like cashews and nutritional yeast, tahini is an easy way to add more protein to a meal. It's also rich in healthy fats. Tahini can bring creaminess to a recipe, as well as a nutty flavor, making it a great addition to curries and stir fries. Tahini is also a perfect base for making salad dressings and glazes. If you have a nut allergy, you can use tahini in place of nuts in lots of recipes.

Avocado

Avocado is another way to enhance creaminess in recipes. With 13 grams of fiber and 4 grams of protein per serving, avocado is as healthy as it is tasty. Use avocado to make a killer chocolate mousse or an indulgent pasta sauce. Add an avocado to a smoothie to make it even creamier.

Flax Seeds

Flax seeds are an easy way to add protein to any meal. Flax seeds are also high in omega fatty acids, which are super-important for radiant skin. Just throw some ground flax seeds into a smoothie for an instant boost. Doctors also recommend adding omega fatty acids to your diet during the winter in conjunction with vitamin D to fight off the winter blues.

As if that weren't enough, these little seeds are also a great egg replacement. Mix a tablespoon of ground flax seeds with a tablespoon of water for an instant egg substitute that you can use in almost any recipe.

Make sure you buy ground flax seeds, because your body is unable to digest them whole.

Cauliflower

Cauliflower is a low-carb replacement for rice, potatoes, and sometimes even flour, making this one of the world's most versatile vegetables. Low in calories, but high in vitamin C, cauliflower is a nutritional win-win. When cooked and blended, cauliflower gets super creamy, making it a perfect nutrient-dense cream replacement. Add to soups and curries in place of heavy cream, or use it to make "cheese."

"Is Being Vegan Expensive?"

Some specialty items might be more expensive, but a vegan diet does not have to be an expensive endeavor. When you go to the grocery store, what's usually more expensive, meat or vegetables?

The best way to save money on a vegan diet is by shopping at local farmers' markets and buying the produce that is in season. Buying from local farmers not only supports your community, it's also more eco-friendly because the produce does not have to be transported long distances.

Check out this guide to seasonal produce.

Fall

Pomegranate, butternut squash, apples, pears, figs, sweet potatoes, arugula, beets, peppers, broccoli, celery, eggplant, cranberries, potatoes, lettuce, mushrooms, limes, pumpkins, green beans, zucchini.

Winter

Beets, cabbage, oranges, Brussels sprouts, onions, clementines, kale, cauliflower, leeks, grapefruit, lemons, mandarin oranges, shallots, radishes, turnips, winter squash, tangerines.

Spring

Asparagus, strawberries, cherries, rhubarb, kumquats, fava beans, apricots, chard, kiwis, new potatoes, peas, spinach, spring onions.

Summer

Basil, avocados, peaches, cantaloupes, blackberries, mangoes, bell peppers, lemongrass, chard, blueberries, okra, chickpeas, melons, collard greens, grapes, cucumbers, figs, plums, raspberries, spinach, watermelons, summer squash, nectarines.

Organic produce is often more expensive than conventional, but it is better for the environment and your body because it does not contain harmful pesticides and other chemicals. That being said, it's not always necessary to eat only organic produce.

Experts have developed lists called the Clean 15 and the Dirty Dozen. The Clean 15 are the 15 fruits and veggies that have the lowest levels of pesticides and are therefore safe to eat even if they aren't organic. The Dirty Dozen are the 12 fruits and vegetables highest in chemicals. You shouldn't eat these unless you can get them organic.

The Clean 15

Corn, pineapple, cauliflower, honeydew, avocado, kiwi, onions, eggplant, cabbage, sweet peas, asparagus, papaya, mangos, cantaloupe, grapefruit.

The Dirty Dozen

Spinach, pears, strawberries, bell peppers, celery, nectarines, potatoes, cherries, apples, grapes, peaches, tomatoes.

"Is Being Vegan A Lot Of Work?"

Being vegan is about as much work as you want it to be. Plenty of vegans consider their diet not just a lifestyle choice but also a hobby. Cooking vegan is fun and requires creativity, so when you see your vegan friends cooking for hours every day, it's probably because they love cooking and eating delicious, healthy meals, not because they have to.

Being a vegan can be easy and low maintenance. Plenty of the recipes in this cookbook don't even require cooking and can be made in 10 minutes or less.

With all of these delicious yet nutritious options, being a vegan is really fun. As an added bonus, vegan food is usually lower in calories, which means you get to eat seemingly decadent meals without harming your health or waistline.

When vegan food can be this healthy, but taste oh so good, why would you ever eat meat or dairy?

Slow Cooker Tips

Keep It Closed
One major mistake people make when using a slow cooker is not properly sealing the lid. Since you'll likely be cooking a meal for several hours, you want to make sure the moisture is trapped to avoid burning the food. Not sealing could also allow steam to spray out and burn your hands!

Preheat
Like your oven, your slow cooker should be preheated before you add the ingredients!

Proper Care
The ceramic dish inside your slow cooker needs to be properly cleaned each time you use it. If any food is stuck to it, soak the pot overnight. The ceramic can actually be quite delicate and prone to cracking if faced with extreme changes in temperature, so do not put it in your slow cooker straight from the refrigerator.

Don't Overfill
Keep in mind that ingredients will likely expand while cooking, which means that the food within your slow cooker can become overcrowded or even spill out.

Know Your Ingredients
Not all ingredients can stand up to long exposure to heat. Some ingredients, like honey, are even said to turn toxic when heated for a long period of time. Ingredients that cannot stand the test of time should be avoided, or added in at the end. For example, pasta

will often turn mushy if cooked for too long. If you're making noodle soup or a pasta dish, add your pasta in at the end and keep an eye on it.

Grease

This one is pretty self explanatory. If you don't grease the inside of your crock pot, you'll probably have to deal with burning and sticking. Not to mention how difficult it will be to clean!

Keep It Fresh

Generally, frozen ingredients don't do well in the slow cooker. Frozen foods tend to cook much faster, without releasing flavors, which defeats the purpose of slow cooking. Frozen butternut squash in particular ends up with a terrible taste and texture.

Consider Alcohol

Alcohol is a great flavor enhancer, especially for slow cooking. Because it is capable of bonding water and fat molecules together, alcohol can bind flavors that usually wouldn't jive. Note that slow cooking will not diminish alcohol content in the same way as regular cooking, so a little goes a long way. This also means you'll only want to use wine you would be willing to drink. Please be sure to keep the higher alcohol content in mind when cooking for those with alcohol issues.

Also consider vanilla extract, which contains alcohol. This won't cook away either, so use only the highest quality vanilla extract.

Breakfast

Vegan Omelet

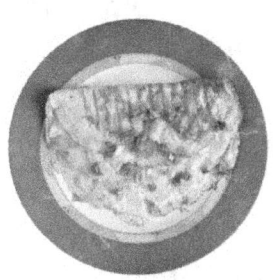

Protein in the morning helps keep you energized throughout the day, so a protein-packed omelet is the perfect way to begin your day. Why should vegans have to miss out?
Yields: 2 servings – Preparation Time: 10 minutes – Cooking Time: 1 hour
Nutrition facts per serving: calories 356, total fat 16 g, carbs 29 g, protein 16 g, sodium 636 mg

Ingredients
1 cup silken tofu
2 cloves garlic
2 tablespoons nutritional yeast
½ teaspoon turmeric
½ teaspoon paprika
½ cup mushrooms, sliced

½ bell pepper, diced
½ tomato, diced
½ cup vegan cheddar
Salt and pepper

Preparation
1. In a food processor, combine tofu, garlic, nutritional yeast, and spices. Pulse until smooth. You may need to add a tablespoon or so of water.
2. Pour mixture into the slow cooker and stir in veggies and cheese.
3. Cook covered on high for an hour or until vegetables and tofu have reached your desired tenderness.

Breakfast Casserole

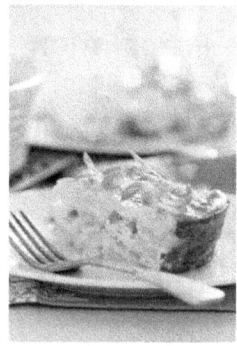

Casseroles are filling meals that are easy to make. This one calls for everything but the kitchen sink, so get creative!

Yields: 4 servings – Preparation Time: 10 minutes – Cooking Time: 6 hours
Nutrition facts per serving: calories 181, total fat 8 g, carbs 25 g, protein 4 g, sodium 281 mg

Ingredients
3 cups hash brown potatoes
1 cup vegan milk
1 onion, diced
1–2 cups veggies of choice
½–1 cup vegan cheddar cheese
1 teaspoon paprika
Salt and pepper

Preparation
1. Combine all ingredients in the slow cooker. Cook covered on low for 6 hours.

Stuffed Apples

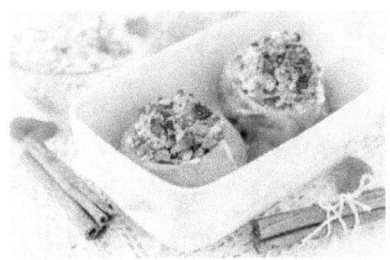

According to Ayurveda, the yogic science of nutrition, eating warm food in the morning helps get your digestion started. That makes these warm, cinnamon-y apples the perfect way to start your day.

Yields: 4 servings – Preparation Time: 10 minutes – Cooking Time: 1½ hours

Nutrition facts per serving: calories 536, total fat 22 g, carbs 78 g, protein 10 g, sodium 221 mg

Ingredients
4 apples
1 cup rolled oats
¼ cup vegan butter
5 tablespoons maple syrup
1½ teaspoons cinnamon
½ teaspoon ground ginger
¼ teaspoon ground cloves
½ cup chopped nuts

Preparation
1. Use a spoon or melon baller to scoop out the insides of the apples.
2. In a large bowl, mix together the chopped nuts, spices, butter, oats, and 2–3 tablespoons of maple syrup. Fill each apple with the mixture.
3. Place the apples in the slow cooker and cover. Cook on high until apples are soft, about 1½ hours.
4. Top with more maple syrup and a dusting of cinnamon and serve warm.

Coffee Cake

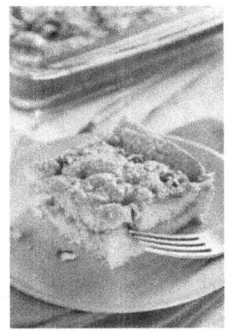

Got a sweet tooth in the morning? This cake is leagues better than eating donuts. Bring it into work to knock the socks off of your co-workers.

Yields: 6 servings – Preparation Time: 10 minutes – Cooking Time: 1½ hours

Nutrition facts per serving: calories 359, total fat 12 g, carbs 57 g, protein 6 g, sodium 88 mg

Ingredients
Cake:
1½ cups flour (oat flour if gluten-free)
½ cup maple syrup
½ cup vegan milk, unsweetened
2 tablespoons vegan butter (or coconut oil)
1 teaspoon baking soda
1 teaspoon vanilla extract
2 flax eggs
Pinch of salt

Topping:
½ cup flour
2 tablespoons brown sugar (or maple syrup)
2 tablespoons vegan butter, solid (or solid coconut oil)
1 teaspoon cinnamon
Optional:
Chopped walnuts

Preparation
1. Mix the ingredients for the topping together until crumbly; set aside.
2. Mix cake batter ingredients together. Line the slow cooker with baking paper (or better yet, slow cooker liner). Add the cake batter and layer the topping on top. Insert a paper towel beneath the lid to collect condensation.
3. Cook on high for 1½ to 2½ hours or until a toothpick comes out clean.
4. Serve warm or store for later.

Crockpot Oatmeal

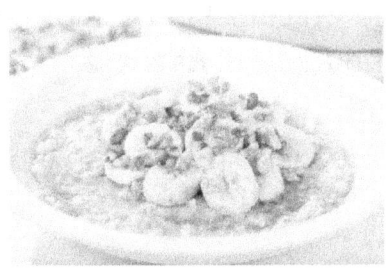

Oatmeal is filling and proven to reduce cholesterol. It also has the perfect balance of protein and carbs to get your day started. This recipe will have everyone saying, "Please, sir, I want some more."

Yields: 6 servings – Preparation Time: 10 minutes – Cooking Time: 6 hours

Nutrition facts per serving: calories 523, total fat 37 g, carbs 49 g, protein 8 g, sodium 88 mg

Ingredients
4 cups vegan milk, unsweetened
1 cup steel cut oats
1–2 bananas, ripe, sliced
½ cup maple syrup
1 teaspoon cinnamon
¼ cup chopped nuts
Optional:
½ cup carob chips
1 tablespoon ground flax seeds
2 tablespoons almond butter

Preparation
1. Oil the sides of the slow cooker. Mix all ingredients (except the carob chips) in the slow cooker. Cook on low for 6–8 hours until oats are tender. Feel free to cook overnight.
2. Serve warm. Top with carob chips, maple syrup, cinnamon, or nut butter.

Breakfast Brownies

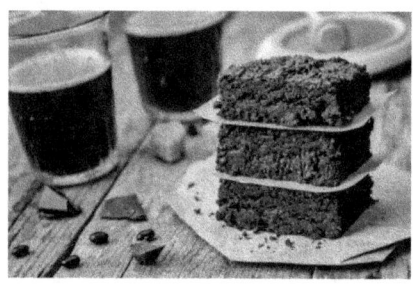

Who says brownies are for dessert? These are filled with protein and healthy fiber, guaranteed to keep you feeling full all morning.

Yields: 9 servings – Preparation Time: 10 minutes – Cooking Time: 6 hours

Nutrition facts per serving: calories 230, total fat 12 g, carbs 28 g, protein 6 g, sodium 552 mg

Ingredients
1 15-ounce can black beans, sodium free, drained and rinsed
1 cup vegan milk
½ cup oat flour
2 flax eggs
¼-½ cup cocoa powder
½ cup maple syrup
¼ cup vegan butter (or coconut oil)
2 teaspoons vanilla extract
1 teaspoon baking soda

Preparation
1. In a food processor or blender, slowly add vegan milk while blending the other ingredients together until completely smooth. You may not need to use all of the milk.
2. Cook on low for 6–8 hours until a toothpick comes out clean.

Beverages

Gingerbread Latte

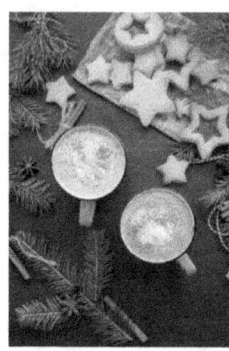

There's nothing like the smell of fresh-baked gingerbread. This recipe makes a big batch, so you can share with your family during the holidays.
Yields: 8 servings – Preparation Time: 5 minutes – Cooking Time: 3 hours
Nutrition facts per serving: calories 365, total fat 36 g, carbs 12 g, protein 4 g, sodium 26 mg

Ingredients
6–8 cups coconut milk (decide based on how strong you like your lattes)
¼ cup maple syrup (or molasses)
2 teaspoons cinnamon, ground
1 teaspoon ginger, ground
½ teaspoon nutmeg, ground
½ teaspoon cloves, ground

3 cups brewed coffee
1 teaspoon vanilla extract
Optional:
⅓ cup pumpkin puree
Coconut whipped cream

Preparation
1. Combine all ingredients in the slow cooker and cook on low, covered, for 2–3 hours. Make sure it doesn't boil. You can then leave the latte on warm setting for 2 hours.
2. Serve warm topped with whipped cream and a dusting of cinnamon.

Peppermint Hot Chocolate

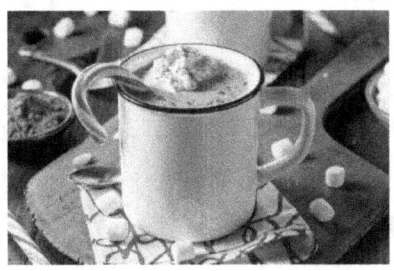

Hot chocolate is a childhood classic. This grownup version is just as tasty (if not more). Add some Kahlua or peppermint schnapps to really amp up your hot chocolate.

Yields: 6 servings – Preparation Time: 5 minutes – Cooking Time: 3 hours

Nutrition facts per serving: calories 355, total fat 33 g, carbs 19 g, protein 4 g, sodium 23 mg

Ingredients
4 cups coconut milk
⅓ cup cocoa powder
⅓ cup maple syrup (or agave nectar)
½ teaspoon peppermint extract

Optional:
Coconut whipped cream
Crushed candy cane

Preparation
1. Mix all ingredients together, then cook covered on low for 3 hours or on high for 1½ hours.
2. Serve immediately or leave on warm setting.

Hot Buttered Rum

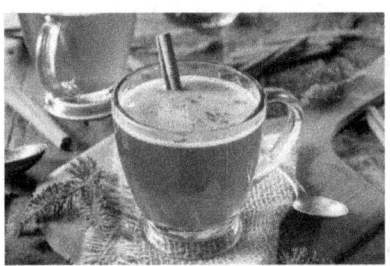

Hot buttered rum is an old school way to warm up on a winter day. Surprise your friends with a vegan take on this classic.

Yields: 10 servings – Preparation Time: 5 minutes – Cooking Time: 6 hours

Nutrition facts per serving: calories 293, total fat 9 g, carbs 29 g, protein 0 g, sodium 105 mg

Ingredients
2 cups brown sugar, unpacked (or maple syrup)
2 cups rum
½ cup vegan butter
2 cups water
3–5 cinnamon sticks
3–6 cloves, whole
1 teaspoon vanilla extract

Optional:
1 teaspoon orange zest
Coconut whipped cream

Preparation
1. Add all ingredients to the slow cooker. If you would like a stronger alcohol content, omit the rum at this point. Stir together, cover, and cook on low for 5–6 hours.
2. Stir in rum, if you haven't already done so, and allow to warm. Serve warm with whipped cream and a dusting of cinnamon.

Horchata Latte

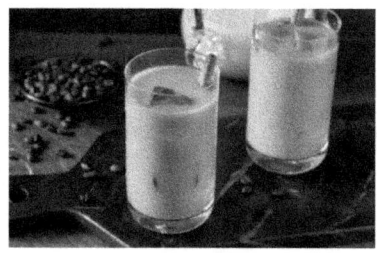

Horchata is perfect for vegans because it's naturally creamy without dairy! This Latin American treat is a great addition to a pool party or beach day.

Yields: 8 servings – Preparation Time: 8 hours – Cooking Time: 4 hours

Nutrition facts per serving: calories 181, total fat 6 g, carbs 29 g, protein 2 g, sodium 6 mg

Ingredients
1 cup rice (long grain white is the most authentic Mexican option; use brown rice for a nutty flavor)
5 cups water, hot
2 tablespoons instant coffee
1 cup coconut milk
2 cinnamon sticks
⅓ cup maple syrup
1 teaspoon vanilla extract

Preparation
1. Mix the hot water, cinnamon, and rice together. Allow to sit overnight or for at least 6 hours.
2. Pour the water-and-rice mixture into the blender and blend until smooth. No need to remove the cinnamon. Strain through a cheesecloth into the slow cooker.
3. Add the maple syrup, coffee, and vanilla. Cook on low for 4 hours.
4. Serve warm, or over ice for a more authentic experience.

Soups

Ginger Carrot Soup

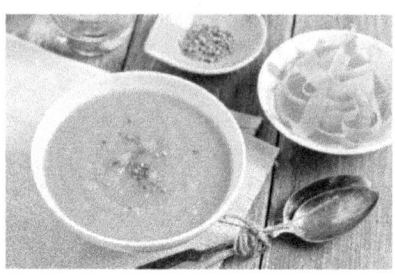

This soup is warm and delicious—plus, ginger is a natural antibiotic perfect for when you're sick. This soup is sure to cure what ails you!

Yields: 4 servings – Preparation Time: 8 hours – Cooking Time: 4 hours

Nutrition facts per serving: calories 220, total fat 12 g, carbs 21 g, protein 3 g, sodium 282 mg

Ingredients
6 carrots, peeled and chopped
1 sweet potato, peeled and chopped
1 onion, diced
4 cups vegetable broth

1 can coconut milk, unsweetened, full fat
1½ teaspoons curry powder
1 tablespoon fresh ginger, peeled and minced
1 clove garlic, minced

Preparation
1. Combine all ingredients in the slow cooker. Cook on low for at least 7 hours, or on high for 3 hours.
2. Use an immersion blender to blend the soup, or pour all ingredients into a traditional blender.
3. Serve warm.

Split Pea Soup

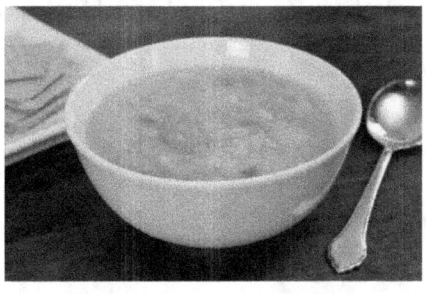

Split pea soup makes for a nutritious addition to any meal. Pair with a salad for the healthiest lunch in town.
Yields: 4 servings – Preparation Time: 15 minutes – Cooking Time: 4 hours
Nutrition facts per serving: calories 272, total fat 1 g, carbs 75 g, protein 25 g, sodium 297 mg

Ingredients

1 pound split peas, rinsed and dried
6 cups vegetable broth
2 carrots, peeled and diced
2 celery stalks, diced
3 cloves garlic, minced
1 onion, diced
1 bay leaf
1 teaspoon cumin
1 teaspoon sage
1 teaspoon thyme
Salt and pepper (to taste)

Preparation
1. Add all ingredients to the slow cooker. Cook covered on low for at least 4 hours.
2. Serve as is, or blend until smooth with an immersion blender.

Corn Chowder

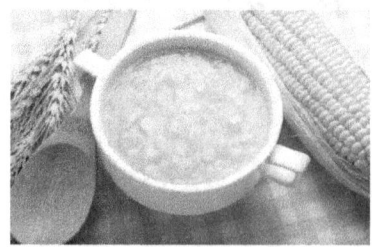

Corn chowder is so creamy and decadent. No reason for vegans to miss out on the flavors of New England.

Yields: 4 servings – Preparation Time: 10 minutes – Cooking Time: 6 hours

Nutrition facts per serving: calories 265, total fat 13 g, carbs 33 g, protein 5 g, sodium 147 mg

Ingredients
2 medium potatoes, washed and chopped
1 onion, chopped
3 cups corn kernels (fresh is better)
2 cloves garlic, minced
1 8-ounce can coconut milk, full fat
4 cups vegetable broth
2 tablespoons vegan butter
1 teaspoon smoked paprika
½ teaspoon red pepper flakes
1 bay leaf
Salt and pepper

Optional:
1 tablespoon cognac

Preparation
1. Add all ingredients to the slow cooker, omitting half of the corn and butter. Cook on low for at least 6 hours, or half that time on high.
2. Use an immersion blender to create a creamy consistency. Add the butter and the rest of the corn

and allow to cook for another 10-15 minutes, or until warmed through.
3. Serve warm. Add hot sauce to taste.

Loaded Baked Potato Soup

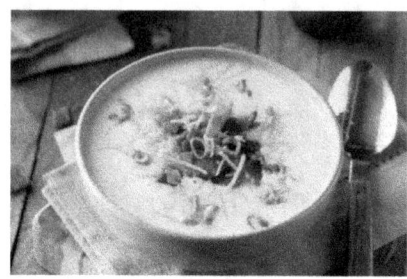

Think soup can't be filling? You'll change your tune after you try this vegan comfort food.
Yields: 4 servings – Preparation Time: 10 minutes – Cooking Time: 8 hours
Nutrition facts per serving: calories 259, total fat 12 g, carbs 33 g, protein 6 g, sodium 152 mg

Ingredients
4–6 medium potatoes
1 onion, chopped
5 cups vegetable broth
½ cup white beans, canned, rinsed
2–3 cloves garlic, minced
2 tablespoons vegan butter
1 cup vegan milk
Salt and pepper

Optional Toppings:
Vegan cheddar
Vegan sour cream
Tempeh bacon
Chives
Hot sauce
Fried onions

Preparation
1. Add all soup ingredients, except for the vegan milk and white beans, to the slow cooker. Cook covered on low for 8 hours or until potatoes are very tender. If you're in a hurry, you can cook on high for 4 hours.
2. Pour in the non-dairy milk and white beans. Heat until warm and creamy, about 10-15 minutes more.
3. Use the immersion blender to create a smooth consistency.
4. Serve with desired toppings.

Homey Tomato Soup

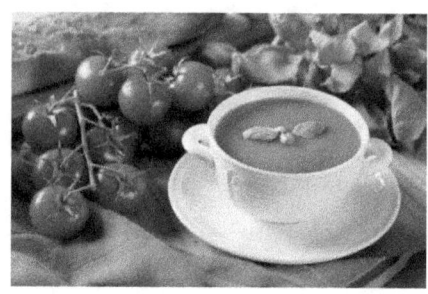

Nothing like Mom's tomato soup and grilled cheese. This one has all the flavor while remaining cruelty free.
Yields: 4 servings – Preparation Time: 10 minutes – Cooking Time: 6 hours
Nutrition facts per serving: calories 284, total fat 9 g, carbs 42 g, protein 10 g, sodium 596 mg

Ingredients
28 ounces diced tomatoes, canned, drained and rinsed
4 cups vegetable stock
½ cup cashews, soaked
½ cup sundried tomatoes
4 cloves garlic, minced
8 ounces tomato paste
1 red pepper, chopped
1 teaspoon oregano
1 teaspoon basil
½ teaspoon red pepper flakes
Salt and pepper

Optional:
Vegan Parmesan
Fresh basil

Preparation
1. Soak the cashews in water as you prep and cook.
2. Add all ingredients, aside from the cashews, to the slow cooker. Cook covered on low for 6 hours.
3. Add the soaked cashews and blend with an immersion blender.
4. Serve warm with desired toppings.

Turmeric Apple Soup

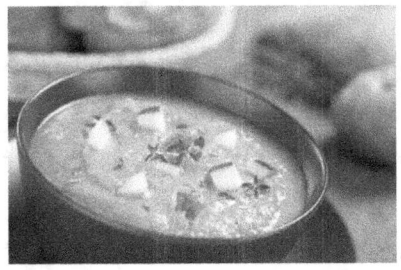

Turmeric has been shown to have countless health benefits. This soup is a delicious way to eat turmeric, and it's also a great way to utilize those fall harvest apples!

Yields: 6 servings – Preparation Time: 10 minutes – Cooking Time: 6 hours

Nutrition facts per serving: calories 255, total fat 13 g, carbs 32 g, protein 4 g, sodium 270 mg

Ingredients
3 medium apples, chopped
2 large sweet potatoes, peeled and chopped
2 cloves garlic
1 onion, diced
1 inch fresh ginger, peeled and minced
½ cup cashews, soaked
4 cups vegetable broth
1 teaspoon turmeric
Salt and pepper

Preparation
1. Add all ingredients, besides the cashews, to the slow cooker. Cook on low for 6 hours or until vegetables are very tender. Soak the cashews while cooking.
2. When the vegetables are ready, add the cashews, then blend until smooth. Season with salt and pepper and serve warm.

Main Courses

Butternut Squash Alfredo

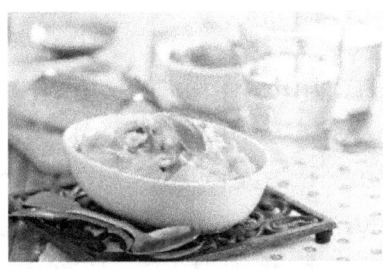

Buttery, complex, and creamy, this pasta elevates comfort food to the realm of gourmet.

Yields: 4 servings – Preparation Time: 10 minutes – Cooking Time: 8½ hours

Nutrition facts per serving: calories 517, total fat 4 g, carbs 104 g, protein 18 g, sodium 127 mg

Ingredients
½ large butternut squash, peeled and cubed
1 onion
¼ cup white wine, dry
2 tablespoons vegan butter
1 teaspoon thyme
3 cups vegetable broth

2 cups dry pasta
Salt and pepper

Optional:
Vegan Parmesan

Preparation
1. Add the butternut squash, wine, garlic, onion, and butter to the slow cooker. Cook on low for 8 hours, stirring and adding vegetable broth as needed.
2. Add the thyme, remaining vegetable broth, and pasta. Cook on high until pasta is tender. This could take up to 30 minutes or more depending on the type of pasta used.

Coconut Curry

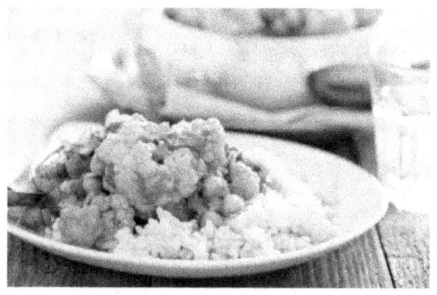

Not only is curry delicious, studies show it may be effective in cancer prevention! All the more reason to add this flavor-filled curry into your life.

Yields: 4 servings – Preparation Time: 10 minutes – Cooking Time: 8½ hours

Nutrition facts per serving: calories 348, total fat 17 g, carbs 41 g, protein 14 g, sodium 632 mg

Ingredients
1 can coconut milk, full fat
2 tablespoons tahini
1 sweet potato, peeled and cubed (or 1 cup butternut squash)
1 16-ounce can chickpeas, drained and rinsed
1 small head cauliflower, cut into florets
4 cloves garlic, minced
1 inch ginger, peeled and shredded
2 tablespoons curry powder
2 tablespoons soy sauce

Preparation
1. Add all ingredients to the slow cooker and cook on high for up to 4 hours, until all vegetables are tender.
2. Serve warm with naan or over quinoa.

Protein-Packed Chili

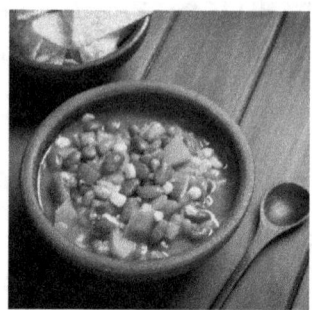

For the days when you need a hearty, protein-packed meal, look no further than this chili. Also perfect for camping trips!
Yields: 4 servings – Preparation Time: 15 minutes – Cooking Time: 8 hours
Nutrition facts per serving: calories 263, total fat 2 g, carbs 51 g, protein 16 g, sodium 702 mg

Ingredients
1 15-ounce can kidney beans, drained and rinsed
1 can black beans, drained and rinsed
1 can chili beans
10 tomatoes, diced
2 onions, diced
2 bell peppers, any color, diced
2 tablespoons chili powder
2 teaspoons cumin
1 teaspoon garlic powder
1 cup dark beer
½ teaspoon cayenne powder

Salt and pepper

Optional toppings:
Jalapeno peppers
Vegan cheddar
Avocado
Vegan sour cream

Preparation
1. Add all ingredients to the crock pot and cook on low for 8 hours.
2. Serve warm with desired toppings.

Masala Lentils

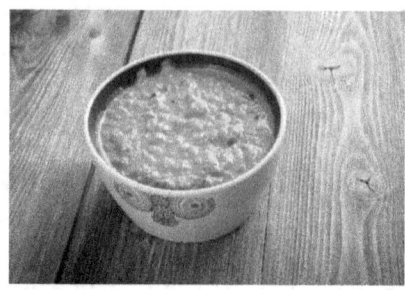

Lentils are filled with iron and protein, so they're a staple every vegan should include in their diet. This Indian inspired version will definitely add some spice to your week.

Yields: 6 servings – Preparation Time: 15 minutes – Cooking Time: 6 hours

Nutrition facts per serving: calories 274, total fat 10 g, carbs 32 g, protein 15 g, sodium 128 mg

Ingredients
2 cups brown lentils, dry
4 cups vegetable broth
1 cup coconut milk, full fat
1 tablespoon vegan butter
4 cloves garlic, minced
1 inch ginger, peeled and shredded
1 tablespoon garam masala
1 teaspoon maple syrup

2 tomatoes, diced

Preparation
1. Add all ingredients to the slow cooker and cook on high for 4 hours or on low for up to 6 hours.
2. Serve warm with naan or over grain.

Tomato Basil Risotto

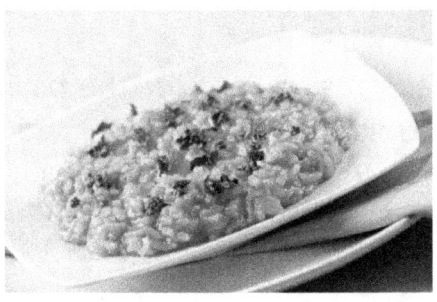

Risotto is a delicious comfort food. Naturally creamy Arborio rice is a vegan secret ingredient.

Yields: 6 servings – Preparation Time: 15 minutes – Cooking Time: 2 hours

Nutrition facts per serving: calories 471, total fat 3 g, carbs 92 g, protein 9 g, sodium 93 mg

Ingredients
1 cup Arborio rice
1 cup white wine, dry

3 cups vegetable broth
¼ cup fresh basil
3 cloves garlic
3 tomatoes, medium, diced
1 tablespoon vegan butter
Salt and pepper

Optional:
Vegan Parmesan

Preparation
1. Add all ingredients, except for the basil and butter, to the slow cooker.
2. Cook on high for 2 hours, or until all liquid has absorbed and rice is tender. Add more liquid as needed.
3. When the rice has finished cooking, add the butter and basil. Mix together and serve warm.

Stuffed Acorn Squash

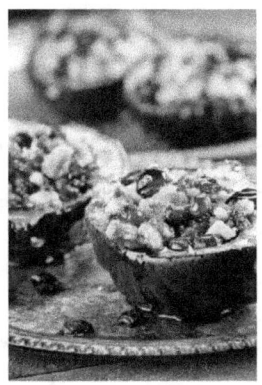

Acorn squash captures the flavors of fall. Take full advantage of the season by serving up this squash in one of its many forms.

Yields: 2 servings – Preparation Time: 15 minutes – Cooking Time: 8 hours

Nutrition facts per serving: calories 532, total fat 21 g, carbs 75 g, protein 13 g, sodium 25 mg

Ingredients
1 acorn squash, cut in half and seeded
1 cup wild rice, cooked
1 cup brown rice, cooked
1 clove garlic, minced
¼ cup white wine
1 tablespoon olive oil
½ cup walnuts, chopped
½ cup pomegranate seeds

2 teaspoons sage, dried
Salt and pepper

Preparation
1. In a large bowl, combine all ingredients, aside from the squash and pomegranate seeds.
2. Stuff the inside of the squash with the mixture.
3. Fill the bottom of the slow cooker with about a half inch of water. Place the squash in the water and slow cook covered and on low for 8 hours. Serve topped with pomegranate seeds.

Vegan Lo-Mein

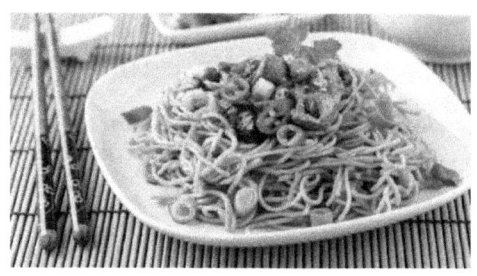

This Chinese inspired dish is healthy, easy to make, and a great way to shake up your weekly meal prep. The veggies listed are just a recommendation; feel free to use whatever you have available.

Yields: 2 servings – Preparation Time: 10 minutes – Cooking Time: 1 hour

Nutrition facts per serving: calories 461, total fat 2 g, carbs 93 g, protein 17 g, sodium 713 mg

Ingredients
3 tablespoons hoisin sauce
2½ tablespoons soy sauce (low sodium preferred)
1 tablespoon maple syrup
1 tablespoon rice vinegar (optional)
3 garlic cloves, minced
1½ tablespoons fresh ginger, peeled and shredded
2 bell peppers
1 carrot, peeled and chopped
½ cup mushrooms
½ cup snow peas
½ cup vegetable broth
3 cups whole wheat linguine noodles, cooked (or rice noodles)

Optional Toppings:
Fried tofu
Edamame

Preparation
1. Add all vegetables, sauces, and broth to the slow cooker. Cook on high for 1 hour, or until vegetables are tender.
2. Add cooked noodles and stir together until warm.

Mushroom Bourguignon

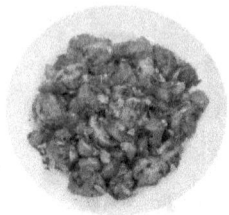

Mushrooms are a nutritional powerhouse and a perfect replacement for beef in vegan recipes. This vegan interpretation of the French gourmet dish is sure to impress.

Yields: 2 servings – Preparation Time: 15 minutes – Cooking Time: 8 hours

Nutrition facts per serving: calories 363, total fat 12 g, carbs 37 g, protein 12 g, sodium 636 mg

Ingredients
1 pound mushrooms, variety, raw (about 4–6 cups)
5 cloves garlic
1 cup red wine, dry
2 tablespoons vegan butter
1 onion, diced
3 tablespoons tomato paste
1 cup mushroom broth
2 carrots, peeled and chopped
1–2 tablespoons flour (optional)

1 teaspoon thyme
Salt and pepper

Preparation
1. Add all ingredients to the slow cooker. Cook covered on low for 5–8 hours. Stir occasionally and add liquid as needed.
2. Once the mushrooms have created a thick sauce, serve over egg noodles or mashed potatoes.

Vegan Stroganoff

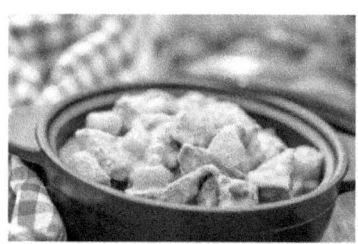

Stroganoff is originally an Eastern European dish, but now there are dozens of different varieties. Try this vegan version for a taste of the Old Country.

Yields: 2 servings – Preparation Time: 15 minutes – Cooking Time: 5 hours

Nutrition facts per serving: calories 379, total fat 16 g, carbs 38 g, protein 16 g, sodium 563 mg

Ingredients
1 10-ounce package "beefless" beef tips
1 onion, diced
3 cloves garlic, minced
2 carrots, peeled and chopped
¼ -½ cup vegan sour cream
1 tablespoon cognac
1 tablespoon vegan butter
1 teaspoon paprika
2 cups vegetable broth

2 tablespoons tomato paste (or ketchup)
1 tablespoon vegan Worcestershire sauce (optional)
1 16-ounce package egg-free egg noodles

Preparation
1. Add all ingredients, EXCEPT the egg noodles, to the slow cooker and stir well. Cook on low for 5 hours.
2. 15-20 minutes before serving, cook egg noodles according to instructions.
3. Serve over cooked egg noodles.

Truffle Oil Mac & Cheese

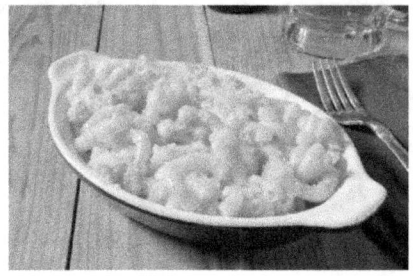

Who says mac & cheese is for kids? Upgrade your mac & cheese with vegan replacements and truffle oil.

Yields: 4 servings – Preparation Time: 10 minutes – Cooking Time: 6 hours

Nutrition facts per serving: calories 400, total fat 19 g, carbs 46 g, protein 18 g, sodium 116 mg

Ingredients
6 ounces dry pasta (elbow macaroni preferred)
1 cup cashews, soaked for at least 6 hours
¼ cup nutritional yeast
1 cup vegan milk, unsweetened
¼ cup white wine (optional)
1 tablespoon truffle oil
2 cups water
Salt and pepper

Preparation
1. In a blender, blend together the cashews, milk, and nutritional yeast until very smooth.
2. Add the cashew mixture to the slow cooker with the rest of the ingredients, omitting the truffle oil, and cook on slow for up to 6 hours until the pasta is cooked. Stir in truffle oil and serve warm.

Veggie Fajitas

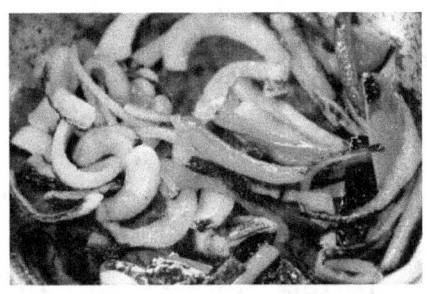

Did you know that one red pepper has more vitamin C than a lemon? Next time you're feeling under the weather, try these easy, healthy fajitas.

Yields: 4 servings – Preparation Time: 10 minutes – Cooking Time: 4 hours

Nutrition facts per serving: calories 201, total fat 4 g, carbs 36 g, protein 6 g, sodium 810 mg

Ingredients
4 flour tortillas
4 bell peppers, any color, sliced
2 onions, sliced
½ lime, juiced
2 teaspoons fajita seasoning
2 cloves garlic, minced
1 tablespoon vegetable oil

Optional toppings:
Guacamole
Salsa
Corn, fresh
Vegan cheddar

Preparation
1. Add veggies to the slow cooker, toss in oil and seasoning. Cook on low for up to 4 hours.
2. Serve on flour tortillas with chosen toppings.

Hearty Meatloaf

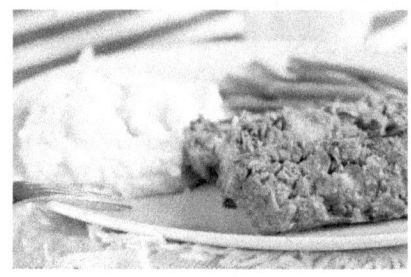

Meatloaf is a hearty American classic you don't have to forget about when you go vegan.

Yields: 4 servings – Preparation Time: 10 minutes – Cooking Time: 4–6 hours

Nutrition facts per serving: calories 343, total fat 11 g, carbs 50 g, protein 14 g, sodium 266 mg

Ingredients
½ cup rolled oats
½ cup cashews, chopped
¼ cup ketchup
1 onion, diced
1 cup carrots, shredded
2 garlic cloves, minced
1½ cups lentils, cooked
1 teaspoon salt
1 teaspoon thyme
2 flax eggs

Preparation
1. Mix everything together in a bowl.
2. Line the slow cooker and fill with the mixture. Shape. Cook on low for 6–8 hours or on high for 4–5 hours.
3. Serve warm with bread, green beans, or mashed potatoes.

Cottage Pie

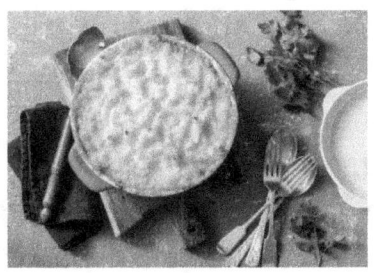

This protein-filled comfort food is sure to delight everybody. Hey, where did the meat go?

Yields: 4 servings – Preparation Time: 10 minutes – Cooking Time: 4–6 hours

Nutrition facts per serving: calories 374, total fat 3 g, carbs 82 g, protein 32 g, sodium 142 mg

Ingredients
3 cups mashed potatoes
1 cup lentils, dry
3 cups vegetable broth
½ cup red wine, dry
2 carrots, peeled and chopped
1 onion, diced
2 cloves garlic, minced
½ cup cauliflower
1 tablespoon tomato paste
1 teaspoon thyme

Preparation
1. Add lentils, veggies, broth, wine, and seasoning to the slow cooker and cook covered on high for 1 hour.
2. Spoon mashed potatoes over the lentils and cook on low for up to 3 hours.
3. Serve warm. Finish with vegan cheddar if desired.

Garlic Spaghetti Squash

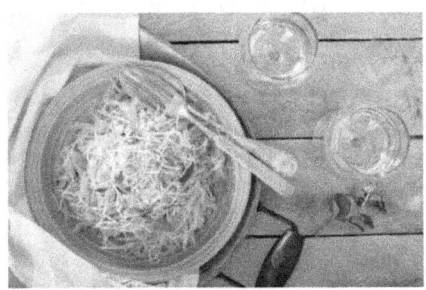

This spaghetti squash is a surefire way to please low-carb and gluten-free friends. This recipe really couldn't be any easier to make.

Yields: 2 servings – Preparation Time: 10 minutes – Cooking Time: 4–6 hours

Nutrition facts per serving: calories 274, total fat 25 g, carbs 25 g, protein 11 g, sodium 733 mg

Ingredients
1 spaghetti squash
½ cup cashews, unsalted
2 tablespoons nutritional yeast
1 teaspoon garlic powder
¼ teaspoon salt
1 tablespoon vegan butter (or olive oil)

Preparation
1. Prick the outside of the spaghetti squash a few times. Fill the bottom of the slow cooker with about an inch of water.
2. Place the whole squash inside and cook for 6 hours on low.
3. While the squash is cooking, add the cashews, salt, nutritional yeast, and garlic powder to the food processor to make a garlic-flavored Parmesan replacement.
4. Slice the squash in half, scoop out the seeds, and shred the insides with a fork.
5. Serve topped with vegan butter and your vegan Parmesan.

Loaded Potatoes

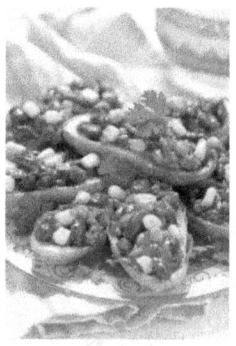

These loaded potatoes are actually a different take on nachos! Packed with flavor and protein.

Yields: 4 servings – Preparation Time: 10 minutes – Cooking Time: 5 hours

Nutrition facts per serving: calories 442, total fat 17 g, carbs 70 g, protein 12 g, sodium 596 mg

Ingredients
4 large potatoes, halved, not peeled
1 cup black beans, cooked
1 cup sweet corn
1 cup vegan cheddar cheese
2 bell peppers, diced
2 tablespoons taco seasoning
2 tablespoons olive oil

Optional toppings:
"Beefless" ground beef
Avocado
Vegan sour cream

Preparation
1. Toss potatoes in olive oil and cook on high for 3 hours, until slightly tender.
2. Fill the center of the potatoes with cheese, beans, corn, peppers, and seasoning. Cook on high for another 2 hours until potatoes are fully cooked and the cheese is melted.
3. Serve with desired toppings.

Vegan Lasagna

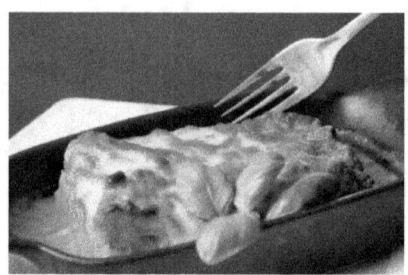

Who doesn't love cheesy lasagna? This version is a perfect option for Meatless Mondays.
Yields: 6 servings – Preparation Time: 10 minutes – Cooking Time: 5 hours

Nutrition facts per serving: calories 577, total fat 24 g, carbs 75 g, protein 16 g, sodium 797 mg

Ingredients
1 24-ounce jar tomato sauce
24 ounces vegan ricotta cheese
½ cup vegan Parmesan cheese
1 eggplant, sliced
1 package lasagna noodles
1 tablespoon olive oil

Preparation
1. Coat the bottom of the slow cooker with tomato sauce and olive oil.
2. Create layers by stacking pasta, ricotta, eggplant, and tomato sauce until you have filled the pot.

Some people like more pasta, others like less, so this is up to you.
3. Top with vegan Parmesan.
4. Cook covered on high for 3 hours. Allow the lasagna to sit after it is done cooking to absorb remaining moisture.

Butternut Dahl

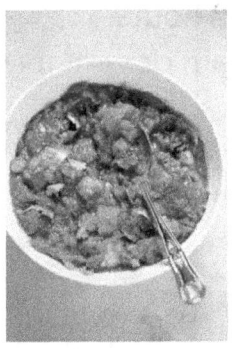

Creamy dhal? Buttery squash? Butternut squash dhal is a match made in heaven.

Yields: 4 servings – Preparation Time: 10 minutes – Cooking Time: 8 hours

Nutrition facts per serving: calories 385, total fat 19 g, carbs 43 g, protein 14 g, sodium 216 mg

Ingredients
1 cup red lentils, dry

2 cups butternut squash, peeled and cubed
2 cloves garlic, minced
2 tablespoons fresh ginger, peeled and minced
1 tablespoon curry powder
1 tablespoon soy sauce, low sodium
2 cups vegetable broth
1½ cups coconut milk, full fat

Preparation
1. Add all ingredients to the slow cooker and cook covered on low for 8 hours.
2. Serve warm over grain or with naan.

White Bean Orzo

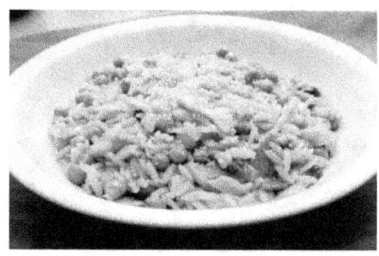

This Mediterranean dish makes for a delightful dinner. Serve leftovers cold the next day for lunch.

Yields: 4 servings – Preparation Time: 10 minutes – Cooking Time: 3 hours

Nutrition facts per serving: calories 495, total fat 7 g, carbs 90 g, protein 20 g, sodium 68 mg

Ingredients
1½ cups orzo pasta, dry
1 cup mushrooms, sliced
½ cup green peas (optional)
3 cups vegetable broth
1 15-ounce can white beans, rinsed and drained
1 onion, diced
2 cloves garlic, minced
2 teaspoons Italian seasoning
2 tablespoons vegan butter
Salt and pepper

Preparation
1. Add all ingredients to the slow cooker, except for the pasta and canned beans. Cook covered on high for 1–2 hours.
2. Add pasta and beans and cook on high for up to 45 minutes, until pasta is tender.

"Butter" Chickpeas

This vegan take on an Indian classic is filled with nutrients that vegans sometimes miss out on.

Yields: 4 servings – Preparation Time: 15 minutes – Cooking Time: 5 hours

Nutrition facts per serving: calories 482, total fat 37 g, carbs 30 g, protein 17 g, sodium 627 mg

Ingredients

1 12-ounce package firm tofu, pressed, cubed
1 15-ounce can chickpeas, drained and rinsed
2 tablespoons vegan butter
1 15-ounce can coconut milk, full fat
1 6-ounce can tomato paste
1 tablespoon fresh ginger, peeled and minced
3 cloves garlic, minced
1 tablespoon curry powder
1 tablespoon garam masala

Preparation

1. Add all ingredients to the slow cooker and cook on low for 5 hours. The sauce should be very thick when it's ready.

Sides

Glazed Brussels Sprouts

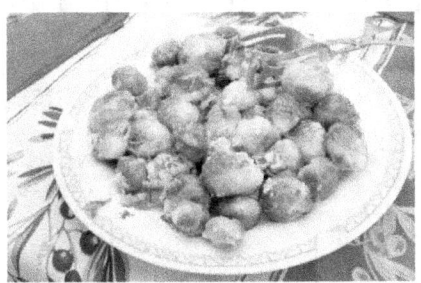

Brussels sprouts aren't for everyone, but this recipe might convince some people to reconsider.

Yields: 4 servings – Preparation Time: 0 minutes – Cooking Time: 2 hours

Nutrition facts per serving: calories 115, total fat 6 g, carbs 14 g, protein 1 g, sodium 77 mg

Ingredients
1 pound Brussels sprouts
⅓ cup balsamic vinegar
2 tablespoons maple syrup
2 tablespoons vegan butter
Salt and pepper

Optional toppings:
Vegan Parmesan

Preparation
1. Add Brussels sprouts to the slow cooker with salt, pepper and butter and cook on high for 1–2 hours.
2. Meanwhile, bring the balsamic vinegar and maple syrup to a boil in a saucepan. Reduce to a simmer and simmer for 8 minutes.
3. Serve Brussels sprouts warm, covered in the balsamic glaze.

Baked Sweet Potatoes

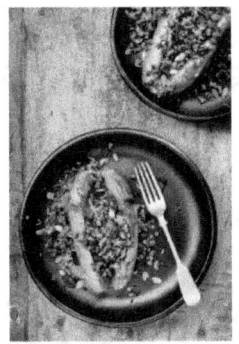

This is a versatile and nutrient-dense side dish. Serve it on Thanksgiving or at a BBQ.

Yields: 4 servings – Preparation Time: 0 minutes – Cooking Time: 4 hours

Nutrition facts per serving: calories 105, total fat 0 g, carbs 24 g, protein 2 g, sodium 280 mg

Ingredients
4 sweet potatoes

Optional toppings:
Vegan butter
Cinnamon
Maple syrup
Stuffing
Salt and pepper

Preparation

1. Wrap the sweet potatoes in aluminum foil. Cook on high for 4 hours.
2. Serve warm with desired toppings.

Jamaican Rice And Beans

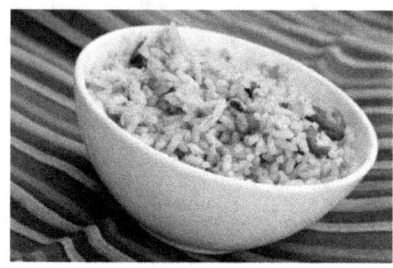

This taste of the Caribbean is an easy way to add more protein to any meal.

Yields: 6 servings – Preparation Time: 0 minutes – Cooking Time: 8 hours

Nutrition facts per serving: calories 329, total fat 16 g, carbs 46 g, protein 10 g, sodium 95 mg

Ingredients
1 15-ounce can coconut milk, full fat
1 cup white rice, dry
1 cup red beans, dry
3 cups vegetable broth
2 limes
1 onion, diced

3 cloves garlic, minced
1 bay leaf
2 teaspoons creole spice
Salt

Preparation
1. Add all ingredients, except for the limes, to the slow cooker and cook covered on low for 8 hours until beans are tender and all liquid has evaporated.
2. Serve with lime juice.

Maple Glazed Carrots

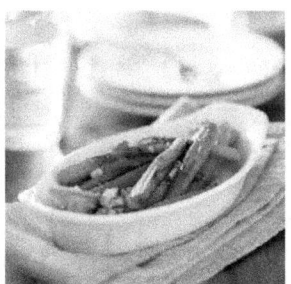

Maple syrup elevates these carrots to a gourmet side perfect with a vegan roast or holiday meal.

Yields: 4 servings – Preparation Time: 10 minutes – Cooking Time: 3 hours

Nutrition facts per serving: calories 180, total fat 11 g, carbs 20 g, protein 0 g, sodium 137 mg

Ingredients

1 pound carrots, peeled and chopped
¼ cup vegan butter
¼ cup maple syrup
1 tablespoon apple cider vinegar
Salt and pepper

Preparation
1. Combine all ingredients in the slow cooker and cook covered on high for 1 hour.
2. Stir.
3. Cook for an additional 2 hours on low.

Stuffed Peppers

You can stuff peppers with just about whatever you have in the pantry, but this recipe is one very tasty combo. Serve this healthy side at a fiesta or picnic.

Yields: 4 servings – Preparation Time: 10 minutes – Cooking Time: 6 hours

Nutrition facts per serving: calories 200, total fat 9 g, carbs 25 g, protein 6 g, sodium 260 mg

Ingredients
4 bell peppers, any color, cored
4 tomatoes, diced
1 onion, diced
1 cup quinoa, cooked

1 cup "beefless" ground beef
1 teaspoon taco seasoning
½ teaspoon paprika

Preparation
1. In a large bowl, combine all ingredients other than the peppers.
2. Stuff each pepper with the mixture. Fill the bottom of the slow cooker with about ¼ to ½ of an inch of water.
3. Cook the peppers on low for 6 hours.

Buttery Mushroom Rice

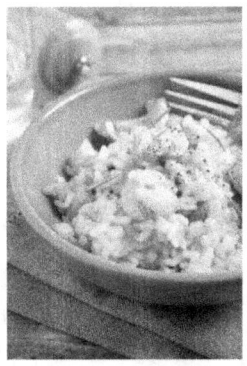

This flavor-filled rice goes great with a vegan roast or grilled veggies.

Yields: 4 servings – Preparation Time: 10 minutes – Cooking Time: 6 hours

Nutrition facts per serving: calories 297, total fat 10 g, carbs 43 g, protein 7 g, sodium 241 mg

Ingredients
½ pound mushrooms, sliced
2 tablespoons vegan butter
1 onion, diced
3 cloves garlic
1 teaspoon thyme
1 cup rice, white
2 cups vegetable broth
½ cup vegan Parmesan

Preparation
1. Add all ingredients to the slow cooker and cook covered on low for 6 hours or on high for half that time.

Snack Mix

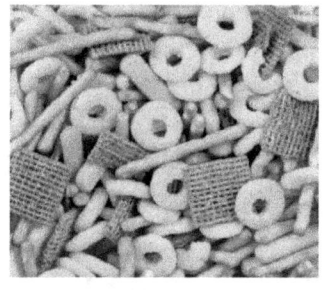

A perfect and easy treat you can bring to any party or throw in a lunchbox in the morning.

Yields: 10 servings – Preparation Time: 0 minutes – Cooking Time: 2 hours

Nutrition facts per serving: calories 84, total fat 3 g, carbs 13 g, protein 2 g, sodium 284 mg

Ingredients
3 cups cereal of your choice (variety recommended)
1 cup mini pretzels
1 cup bagel chips
2 tablespoons vegan butter
½ teaspoon garlic powder
½ teaspoon onion powder
¼ teaspoon paprika
½ teaspoon salt

Preparation
1. Pour cereal, pretzels, and bagel chips into the slow cooker.
2. In a separate bowl, melt butter and mix together with seasonings. Pour over cereal mixture.
3. Cook on high for 2 hours, uncovered.
4. Eat right away or store in an airtight container.

Southern Style Green Beans

This nutrient-dense, protein-filled side goes great with traditional American food and holiday meals. Enjoy it at home or bring to a summer BBQ.

Yields: 4 servings – Preparation Time: 0 minutes – Cooking Time: 3 hours

Nutrition facts per serving: calories 41, total fat 0 g, carbs 7 g, protein 4 g, sodium 67 mg

Ingredients
6 slices tempeh bacon
1 pound fresh green beans
½ onion, diced
½ cup vegetable broth
1 teaspoon thyme
Salt and pepper

Preparation
1. Add all ingredients to the slow cooker and cook covered on high for 3 hours, until green beans are tender.

Cajun Potatoes

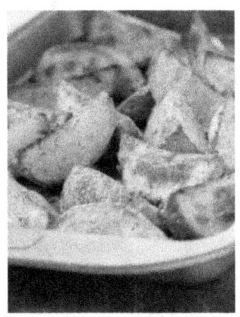

Channel the flavors of New Orleans into everyone's favorite carb.

Yields: 4 servings – Preparation Time: 0 minutes – Cooking Time: 3 hours

Nutrition facts per serving: calories 294, total fat 4 g, carbs 45 g, protein 2 g, sodium 365 mg

Ingredients
3 potatoes, cubed or wedged
4 links vegan sausage, sliced
1 cup corn
½ cup vegetable broth
1–2 teaspoons Cajun seasoning
½ teaspoon red pepper flakes
Salt and pepper

Preparation

1. Add all ingredients to the slow cooker. Cook on low for 7 hours, until potatoes are tender.

Desserts

Apple Nachos

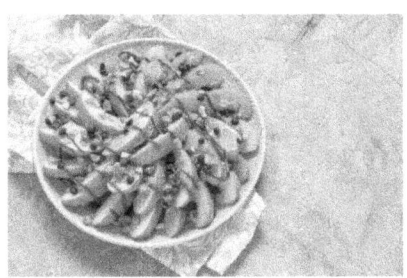

These dessert nachos are a brilliant way to trick your kids into eating fruit.

Yields: 4 servings – Preparation Time: 10 minutes – Cooking Time: 3 hours

Nutrition facts per serving: calories 193, total fat 6 g, carbs 34 g, protein 0 g, sodium 65 mg

Ingredients
4 apples, sliced
2 tablespoons vegan butter
1 teaspoon cinnamon
½ teaspoon ginger
2 tablespoons brown sugar

Optional toppings:

Maple syrup
Caramel sauce
Nut butter
Carob chips
Raisins
Vegan marshmallows

Preparation
1. Place ingredients in the slow cooker and cook covered on low for 3 hours, or until apples have reached your desired tenderness.
2. Finish with desired toppings.

Chai Tea Pie

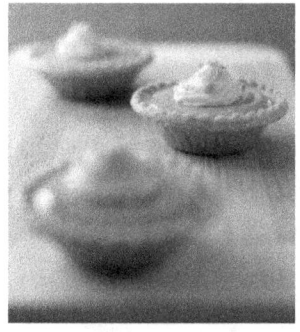

The warm flavors of this pie make a uniquely delicious treat. Bring it to a holiday party for a real knockout.

Yields: 6 servings – Preparation Time: 0 minutes – Cooking Time: 8 hours

Nutrition facts per serving: calories 347, total fat 24 g, carbs 33 g, protein 3 g, sodium 155 mg

Ingredients
1 15-ounce can coconut milk, full fat
¼-½ cup maple syrup (to taste)
1 tablespoon cinnamon
6 cloves
6 cardamom pods
1 teaspoon ground ginger
2 tablespoons flour
1 pie crust (or 6 mini pie crusts)

Preparation
1. Add the coconut milk and spices to the slow cooker. Cook covered on low for 6 hours, stirring occasionally.
2. Remove the cardamom pods and cloves. Slowly stir in flour until the coconut milk thickens. Add the maple syrup. Cook covered on low for up to 2 more hours, until the milk has thickened once more.
3. Pour the mixture into a pie crust and refrigerate for 45 minutes.

Hot Fudge Cake

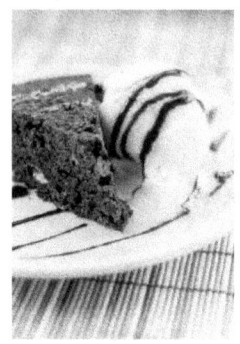

Who says vegans can't eat gooey, decadent chocolate cake? Perfect for a summer picnic.

Yields: 12 servings – Preparation Time: 5 minutes – Cooking Time: 3 hours

Nutrition facts per serving: calories 349, total fat 13 g, carbs 57 g, protein 4 g, sodium 90 mg

Ingredients
2 cups maple syrup
2 flax eggs
2 cups flour
¾ cup cocoa powder
1 cup vegan milk
½ cup vegan butter (or coconut oil)
1 tablespoon baking powder
2 teaspoons vanilla extract

1 cup water (as needed)

Preparation
1. Combine all ingredients in a large bowl, whisking together and adding water as needed.
2. Grease the inside of the slow cooker and pour in the batter.
3. Cook covered on low for 3 hours until cake has set. Use a toothpick to determine when it is ready.

Pumpkin Butter

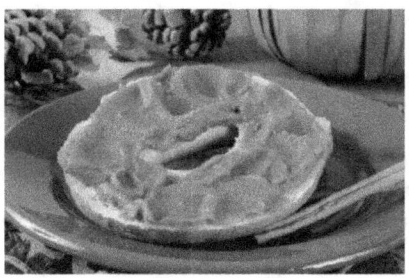

Pumpkin butter is a fall classic that's high in vitamin A. Eat this on a bagel or use it to make frosting!

Yields: 32 servings – Preparation Time: 0 minutes – Cooking Time: 6 hours

Nutrition facts per serving: calories 25, total fat 0 g, carbs 6 g, protein 0 g, sodium 1 mg

Ingredients
1 15-ounce can pumpkin puree
½ cup maple syrup
¼ cup brown sugar
2 tablespoons pumpkin pie spice mix
½ teaspoon vanilla extract

Preparation
1. Mix all ingredients together in the slow cooker. Cook covered on low for up to 6 hours. Stir regularly to prevent burning and sticking.
2. Store in a jar in the refrigerator for up to 2 weeks.

Rosewater Yogurt

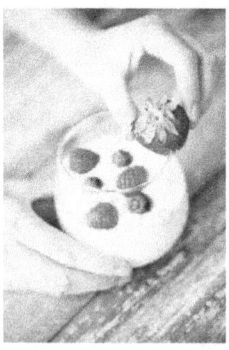

Dessert doesn't have to be filled with sugar and calories. This vegan yogurt will certainly satisfy your sweet tooth nonetheless.

Yields: 4 servings — Preparation Time: 0 minutes — Cooking Time: 10½ hours

Nutrition facts per serving: calories 80, total fat 3 g, carbs 11 g, protein 0 g, sodium 115 mg

Ingredients
4 cups soy or coconut milk
1 tablespoon rosewater
½ cup vegan yogurt or vegan yogurt starter

For serving
Mixed berries
Sweetener

Preparation
1. Place the milk in the slow cooker and cook on low for about 2½ hours. Remove from heat, but leave covered.
2. After the milk sits for 2 hours, stir in the vegan yogurt or starter.
3. Wrap the crock pot in a towel and allow the yogurt to cool for 8 hours in the oven (turned off).
4. The longer the yogurt sits, the sourer and firmer it will become.
5. Stir in rosewater, fruit, and any desired sweetener. Store in the refrigerator.

Poached Pears

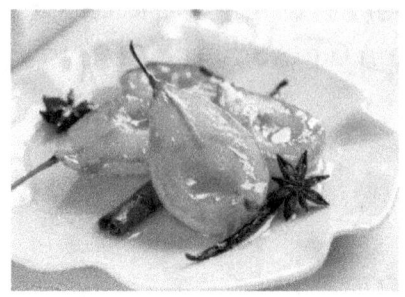

When it comes to dessert, pears are seriously underrated. Serve these as a fall favorite or with ice cream at a summer picnic.

Yields: 8 servings – Preparation Time: 10 minutes – Cooking Time: 6 hours

Nutrition facts per serving: calories 147, total fat 3 g, carbs 32 g, protein 0 g, sodium 36 mg

Ingredients
4 pears, halved, cored, and peeled
1 cup brown sugar, unpacked
2 tablespoons vegan butter
1 tablespoon cinnamon
1 teaspoon ground ginger
1 whole star anise

Preparation

1. Mix all ingredients together in the slow cooker.
2. Cook on low, covered, for up to 6 hours, until pears are tender.

Part 2

Introduction

A vegan diet contains foods of a vegetable nature only. Following this diet, you'll consume grains, nuts, fruits, beans, legumes, and of course, vegetables. Like vegetarianism, it can be a very healthy way to eat. Veganism does differ from vegetarianism, though, in both the foods allowed in the diet, and the reasons behind it.

Vegetarians don't eat meat, either because they don't like it, for health reasons, or because they protest the consumption of animals. Vegans don't eat meat, either – or **any** food from animals, including dairy and eggs. In fact, vegans often don't like to be lumped in with vegetarians, because their motivations are ethical in nature.

Vegans are opposed to the slaughter of animals, certainly. But they also recognize that there is killing involved in the dairy industry as well (male calves are often taken at birth, and either culled or sold for veal). Additionally, animals raised as food are often subject to poor (many would say cruel) living conditions. Vegans oppose these practices.

Additionally, vegans often realize that their way of eating is better for the environment. There is a lot of deforestation taking place to make room for farming, much of it soy, most of which goes to feed the animals we eat. Massive quantities of grain go to these animals, while in other countries, people are starving. So there are human rights aspects to this lifestyle, as well.

Naturally, vegans don't use other animal products either (like leather, for instance), and they oppose animal testing for any reason.

Many of these concerns have never occurred to the average consumer, and on their own they are compelling. However, there are advantages for your body, as well.

1. A vegan diet is richer in certain nutrients. Whole-food vegan diets are generally higher in certain nutrients. However, you do need to make sure you get all the nutrients your body needs. It's advisable to speak with a doctor or nutritionist, to make sure you know how to replace the proteins you'll be eliminating.
2. A vegan diet can help you lose excess weight. Vegan diets have a natural tendency to reduce your calorie intake. This makes them effective at promoting weight loss without the need to actively focus on cutting calories.
3. Veganism appears to lower blood sugar levels and improve kidney function. Vegan diets may reduce the risk of developing type 2 diabetes. They are also particularly effective at reducing blood sugar levels and may help prevent further health problems from developing.
4. Veganism is linked to a lower risk of heart disease. Vegan diets may benefit heart health by significantly reducing the risk factors that contribute to heart disease, such as saturated fat.

5. A vegan diet can reduce pain from arthritis. Vegan diets based on probiotic-rich whole foods can significantly decrease the symptoms of osteoarthritis and rheumatoid arthritis, because vegan foods would tend to discourage the inflammation that causes the pain.

If you're following a vegan lifestyle, you may know these things already. In that case, you're probably also familiar with the amount of work that goes into eating so carefully. That brings us to the topic of slow cookers.

The Benefits Of Using A Slow Cooker

1. Slow cookers can be very convenient. Slow cookers are not just for cooking meat. Vegans work and have families, too – and wouldn't you like to come home to a meal that is all ready to go?
2. Slow cookers save energy. Slow cookers consume much less energy than an electric oven. Your standard oven uses about 4,000 watts per hour. On the other hand, slow cookers consume only 300 watts.
3. The meals are super easy to make. Anyone can master slow cooker meals, because almost all the ingredients in the recipes are added at the same time. You may need to jiggle it to distribute the liquid and spices, but that's it. Put on the lid and

leave it on. The kitchen cover seals in the moisture and the flavor.
4. Slow cookers are very safe to use. Slow cookers are designed to be left unattended. Their maximum power is 300 watts, equivalent to the operation of three 100-watt incandescent bulbs. It is almost impossible to burn your food, and so as long as the wires aren't frayed, they're very safe. Since the ovens are well covered, there is little risk that the food will dry out and burn, which can be a problem when using the oven.
5. Cooking at lower heat is healthier. We recognize that vegetables are healthiest when they're raw. But if we don't want raw food all the time, steaming, poaching, and slow cooking are the healthiest ways to cook not only for food.

Breakfast Recipes

Peach Granola Crumble

A quick and easy recipe for a vegan peach crumble that you can prepare in your slow cooker. It's a healthy breakfast.

Serves 6 – Preparation time 15 minutes – Cooking time 3 hours

Ingredients
4 peaches
4 tablespoons vegan butter, melted, divided
½ cup peach juice
¼ cup agave nectar
2 cups granola, your favorite kind
2 teaspoons ground cinnamon
1 teaspoon ground nutmeg

Preparation
1. Peel and slice the peaches. In a large mixing bowl, toss them with 2 tablespoons melted vegan butter, the peach juice, and agave nectar.
2. Arrange the mixture in the bottom of a slow cooker.
3. In the same mixing bowl, stir together the granola, the remaining butter, ground cinnamon, and ground nutmeg.
4. Sprinkle the topping over the peach slices.

5. Cover the slow cooker and cook on HIGH for 3 hours. Remove the lid, turn off the slow cooker, and let the crisp cool.
6. Serve warm.

Nutrition facts per serving
Calories 232, total fat 4 g, carbs 46.5 g, protein 5.5 g, Sodium 32.2 mg, sugar 1.1 g

Healthy Breakfast Casserole

This is the perfect vegan breakfast to feed a crowd. Whether for a holiday or a casual Saturday, you will love this vegan, simmered breakfast that you can set up overnight.

Serves 4 – Preparation time 15 minutes – Cooking time 4 hours

Ingredients
1 cup tofu
½ cup milk
1 tablespoon ground mustard
¼ teaspoon garlic salt
½ teaspoon salt
¼ teaspoon pepper
1 (15-ounce) bag frozen hash browns
¼ onion, roughly chopped
1 bell pepper, roughly chopped
½ small head of broccoli, roughly chopped
6 ounces vegan cheddar cheese (optional)

Preparation
1. In a blender, combine the tofu and milk, and purée until smooth.
2. In a medium-sized bowl, whisk together the tofu purée, mustard, garlic salt, salt, and pepper. Set aside.
3. Lightly grease the bottom of your slow cooker. Place half the hash browns on the bottom. Layer with chopped onion, bell peppers, broccoli, and vegan cheese (if using). Add the rest of the hash browns, then top with the rest of the onion, bell peppers, broccoli, and cheese. Pour the purée mixture on top.
4. Cover the slow cooker and cook for 4 hours on LOW. After 4 hours, turn off the slow cooker, and remove the lid carefully.
5. Serve hot!

Nutrition facts per serving
Calories 220, total fat 11.2 g, carbs 19.5 g, protein 22.1 g,
Sodium 735 mg, sugar 1.9 g

Overnight Millet And Oats

This healthy millet and oats pot is very tasty! With dates and apples, this is a new twist on oatmeal.

Serves 6 – Preparation time 5 minutes – Cooking time 7 hours

Ingredients
½ cup millet
1 ½ cups steel cut oats (no substitutes)
4 ½ cups almond milk
4 tablespoons brown sugar
2 tablespoons real maple syrup
¼ teaspoon salt
1 ½ teaspoons vanilla extract
¼ cup apples, finely chopped
¼ cup dates, pitted and chopped
Optional: ¼ teaspoon ground cinnamon, fresh berries, splash of almond or soy milk, Additional sugar for topping

Preparation
1. Spray your slow cooker with non-stick spray.
2. Place the millet in a mesh sieve, and rinse well.
3. Combine the rinsed millet, steel cut oats, almond milk, brown sugar, maple syrup, salt, and vanilla extract in the slow cooker. Add the apples and dates, and any other desired toppings.
4. Stir well, and set the slow cooker on LOW.
5. Cook for 6–7 hours.
6. After 7 hours, turn off the slow cooker. Ladle it into serving dishes, and garnish with additional toppings if desired.

Nutrition facts per serving
Calories 251, total fat 3.1 g, carbs 47.7 g, protein 13.4 g,
Sodium 175 mg, sugar 15.9 g

Chia Seed Energy Bar Recipe

Serves 4 – Preparation time 10 minutes – Cooking time 4 hours

Ingredients
1 tablespoon almond butter
1 tablespoon maple syrup
½ cup unsweetened vanilla almond milk
Pinch of salt
1 banana
¼ teaspoon cinnamon
3 tablespoons chia seed
¼ cup raisins
3 tablespoons roasted almonds, roughly chopped
3 tablespoons dried apples, roughly chopped

Preparation
1. Spray a 5-quart slow cooker with cooking spray and cut a piece of parchment to fit the bottom.
2. Mix the almond butter and maple syrup in a large bowl and microwave for about 30 seconds, until the almond butter is melted and creamy.

3. Add the almond milk and salt, and beat until the milk is well incorporated.
4. Mash the banana until well blended and add it to the almond butter mixture, together with the cinnamon, chia seed, raisins, almonds, and dried apple. Mix thoroughly.
5. Pour the mixture into the slow cooker and cook on LOW until the top of the bars is firm, about 4 hours.
6. Carefully remove the bars from the slow cooker. Put them in the refrigerator to cool completely.
7. Cut into your choice of shape, and serve. Leftovers can be stored in an airtight container, or frozen.

Nutrition facts per serving
Calories 350, total fat 10 g, carbs 70 g, protein 5 g, Sodium 255 mg, sugar 25 g

Vegan Pumpkin Spice Syrup

Serves 4 – Preparation time 10 minutes – Cooking time 7 hours

Ingredients
2 cans full-fat coconut milk
2 cups packed light brown sugar
2 cups organic pumpkin purée
1 teaspoon ground cinnamon
1 teaspoon ground ginger
¼ teaspoon ground cardamom
¼ teaspoon ground allspice

Pinch of cloves

Preparation
1. In your slow cooker, combine the coconut milk, brown sugar, pumpkin puree , cinnamon, ground ginger, ground cardamom , ground allspice and cloves. Mix well with a whisk, and cook on LOW for 7 hours.
2. When the cooking time is up, use a whisk to thoroughly mix all the ingredients and break the pieces that are still in the syrup.
3. Keeps in the refrigerator for up to 1 week.

Nutrition facts per serving
Calories 33, total fat 0 g, carbs 7 g, protein 0 g,
Sodium 0 mg, sugar 5 g

Apple Crumble Breakfast Pudding

Serves 6 – Preparation time 10 minutes – Cooking time 4 hours

Ingredients
Pudding
1 cup almond milk
2 cups water
2 tablespoons maple syrup
½ cup chia seeds
2 tablespoons cornstarch
1 teaspoon ground cinnamon

1 pinch salt
5 large apples, sliced – do not peel!

Cinnamon Crunch Topping
½ cup blanched almond flour
¼ cup unsweetened shredded coconut
¼ cup coconut sugar
1 teaspoon cinnamon
¼ cup unsweetened apple sauce
1 teaspoon pure vanilla extract

For serving: raisins, nuts, almond milk

Preparation
1. Mix the almond milk, water, maple syrup, chia seeds, cornstarch, cinnamon, and salt in the bottom of your 3-quart crock pot.
2. Arrange the cut apples on top, and do not combine them.
3. Mix the crunch topping ingredients in a large bowl. Sprinkle them on top of the apples. Cook on LOW for 2–4 hours.
4. Turn off the slow cooker, and let it stand for an hour, uncovered.
5. Garnish with raisins, nuts, and almond milk if desired. Enjoy!

Nutrition facts per serving
Calories 363, total fat 21.5 g, carbs 49.3 g, protein 3.8 g,

Sodium 157 mg, sugar 35 g

Bean And Grain Recipes

Baked Beans

Delicious homemade beans that can be served as a main course. Especially ideal for lazy Sundays or frozen for later.
Serves 4 – Preparation time 15 minutes – Cooking time 8 hours

Ingredients
1 ½ cups of dried white navy beans, soaked overnight
1 teaspoon salt
3 sundried tomatoes, cut in narrow strips
1 large onion, chopped
4 cups water
½ cup ketchup
¼ cup brown sugar, packed
2 tablespoons molasses
1 teaspoon dry mustard

Preparation
1. Drain the soaked beans, and add them to the slow cooker with the salt, sundried tomatoes, onion, and water.

2. Cover the slow cooker, and simmer on HIGH for 5–6 hours, or until tender. Add more water if the mixture begins to dry out
3. Combine the ketchup, brown sugar, molasses, and mustard in a bowl. Pour over the beans and mix.
4. Continue cooking on LOW for 1–2 hours.

Nutrition facts per serving
Calories 193, total fat 0.7 g, carbs 35.9 g, protein 7.8 g, Sodium 84 7mg, sugar 5.9 g

Vegan Chili

All-time favorite for vegans. This recipe is loaded with sweet potatoes, bell peppers, and a variety of beans.

Serves 2 – Preparation time 20 minutes – Cooking time 8 hours

Ingredients
½ medium red onion, chopped
½ green bell pepper, chopped
2 garlic cloves, chopped
½ tablespoon chili powder
½ tablespoon ground cumin
1 teaspoon unsweetened cocoa powder
⅛ teaspoon ground cinnamon
1 teaspoon kosher salt
¼ teaspoon black pepper
½ (28-ounce) can fire roasted tomatoes, diced

½ (15.5-ounce) can black beans, rinsed
½ (15.5-ounce) can kidney beans, rinsed
1 medium sweet potato
1 cup water
For serving: sour cream, scallions, chopped cilantro, and tortilla chips

Preparation
1. In a 4- to 6-quart slow cooker, combine the onion, bell pepper, garlic, chili powder, cumin, cocoa, cinnamon, salt, and black pepper. Add the tomatoes (and their liquid), beans, sweet potato, and water.
2. Cover and cook on LOW for 7–8 hours, until the potatoes are tender and the liquid has thickened.
3. Serve with sour cream, scallions, cilantro, and tortilla chips

Nutrition facts per serving
Calories 174, total fat 2 g, carbs 35 g, protein 7 g, Sodium 834 mg, sugar 7g

Red Beans And Rice

This is a traditional recipe that everyone loves, and it's made easy in the slow cooker!

Serves 4 – Preparation time 15 minutes – Cooking time 8 hours

Ingredients

3 cups water
8 ounces dry kidney beans
1 onion, chopped
½ green bell pepper, chopped
½ stalk celery, chopped, or to taste
2 cloves garlic, minced, or to taste
1 bay leaf
Salt and pepper to taste
Hot cooked rice, for serving

Preparation
1. Combine the water, kidney beans, onion, green bell pepper, celery, garlic, and bay leaf in the bowl of a slow cooker and stir to combine. Set the slow cooker to LOW, and cook for at least 8 hours. Remove and discard the bay leaf.
2. Meanwhile, cook the rice according to the package directions. Serve with the red bean mixture.
3. Season with salt and ground black pepper to taste.

Nutrition facts per serving
Calories 286.5, total fat 9.7 g, carbs 42 g, protein 16.5 g,
Sodium 322 mg, sugar 1.7 g

Three-Bean Vegan Chili

This vegan chili is a perfect blend of vegetables, spices, and protein-packed beans.

Serves 4 – Preparation time 15 minutes – Cooking time 8 hours

Ingredients
2 tablespoons vegetable oil
1 onion, finely diced
1 red bell pepper, finely diced
1 green bell pepper, finely diced
1 jalapeño pepper, seeded and minced
2 cloves garlic, minced
¼ teaspoon salt
1 tablespoon chili powder
1 teaspoon ground cumin
1 teaspoon dried oregano
2 tablespoons tomato paste
½ (28-ounce) can diced tomatoes
1 ¾ cups water
½ (15.5-ounce) can black beans
½ (15.5-ounce) can kidney beans
½ (15.5-ounce) can chickpeas
Fresh cilantro leaves (optional)

Preparation
1. Coat the bowl of a 6-quart slow cooker with the oil. Add the onion, bell peppers, jalapeño, garlic, and salt, and stir to combine. Add the chili powder, cumin, oregano, tomato paste, tomatoes, and water.
2. Cover, and cook on LOW for 4 hours.

3. Drain and rinse the beans and add them to the cooker, stirring to combine. Cover and cook on LOW for another 2–4 hours.
4. Top each serving with cilantro.

Nutrition facts per serving
Calories 245, total fat 2.9 g, carbs 45.1 g, protein 12.9 g,
Sodium 855 mg, sugar 4.8 g

Spicy Chipotle Black-Eyed Peas

Black-eyes peas are the perfect comfort food, and this healthy recipe only takes a little while to make!

Serves 6 – Preparation time 20 minutes – Cooking time 8 hours

Ingredients
1 tablespoon olive oil
½ tablespoon balsamic vinegar
½ cup red bell pepper, chopped
½ cup celery, chopped
½ cup carrot, chopped
½ cup onion, chopped
1 teaspoon garlic, minced
1 (16-ounce) package dry black-eyed peas
2 cups water
2 teaspoons vegetable bouillon base
1 teaspoon ground cumin

½ teaspoon ground black pepper

Preparation
1. Heat the olive oil and balsamic vinegar in a pan. Sauté the red pepper, celery, carrot, onion, and garlic in the hot oil until the onion is transparent, 5–8 minutes.
2. Transfer the mixture to a slow cooker. Stir in the peas, water, and vegetable base, and stir. Add the cumin and black pepper.
3. Cook in the slow cooker over LOW until the black-eyed peas are very tender and the flavors mix, about 8 hours.

Nutrition facts per serving
Calories 245, total fat 2.9 g, carbs 45.1 g, protein 12.9 g,
Sodium 855 mg, sugar 4.8 g

Wild Rice Medley

This wild rice mix recipe with pine nuts is easy to prepare in a slow cooker. Grains, nuts and vegetables combine to give this dish a wonderful texture.

Serves 6 – Preparation time 20 minutes – Cooking time 5 hours

Ingredients
1 cup uncooked wild rice

⅓ cup celery, chopped
1 tablespoon olive oil
1 teaspoon fresh thyme
¼ teaspoon salt
⅛ teaspoon pepper
1 cup onion, chopped
1 cup carrots, chopped
1 ½ cups vegetable broth
3 tablespoons pine nuts
¼ cup dried cherries, chopped
Fresh parsley, chopped, if desired

Preparation
1. Spray a slow cooker with cooking spray. Combine the wild rice, chopped celery, olive oil, thyme, salt, pepper, onion, carrots, and vegetable broth in the slow cooker.
2. Cover the slow cooker and cook on LOW for 5–6 hours, or until the rice is tender and the liquid has been absorbed.
3. In the meantime, sprinkle the pine nuts in a large pan. Cook over medium heat for 5–7 minutes, stirring frequently, until the nuts are golden brown. Set them aside.
4. Just before serving, mix the cherries and the roasted pine nuts with the wild rice. Sprinkle with parsley.

Nutrition facts per serving
Calories 375, total fat 5.0 g, carbs 51.1 g, protein 34.5 g,

Sodium 714.3 mg, sugar 4.8 g

Barley And Bean Tacos With Avocado Chipotle Cream

Make these tacos easily in the slow cooker. Full of barley, beans, and many vegetables, the avocado cream makes them memorable.

Serves 4 – Preparation time 15 minutes – Cooking time 6 hours

Ingredients
For the filling:
½ red onion, chopped
½ cup frozen corn
½ can black beans, drained and rinsed
½ (14-ounce) can fire-roasted diced tomatoes
½ cup barley
1 cup vegetable broth
Wedge of lime
½ teaspoon cumin
¼ teaspoon smoked paprika
¼ teaspoon salt
¼ teaspoon garlic powder

For the avocado chipotle cream:
½ ripe avocado

1 tablespoon plain Greek yogurt
1 teaspoon chipotle pepper in adobo sauce, minced
Pinch of salt, or more to taste

For serving:
Flour or corn tortillas
Cilantro, chopped
Feta, crumbled

Preparation
1. To make the filling, **combine all the filling ingredients in a slow cooker. Stir well, cover, and simmer for 5–6 hours, until most of the liquid is absorbed and the barley is tender and chewy.**
2. **To make the avocado chipotle cream**, remove the avocado pit and scoop the flesh into a medium bowl. Mash it well with a fork. Add the Greek yogurt, chopped chipotle, and salt. Mix until well blended.
3. To serve, **spoon some of the filling into a tortilla. Garnish with avocado cream, cilantro, and feta.**

Nutrition facts per serving
Calories 219.8, total fat 5.8 g, carbs 34 g, protein 9.9 g, Sodium 18.8 mg, sugar 0.2 g

Slow Cooker Almond Quinoa Curry

This quinoa curry with almonds is one of the easiest foods to prepare. Just throw all the ingredients in the slow cooker, and let it cook.

Serves 4 – Preparation time 15 minutes – Cooking time 4 hours

Ingredients
1 cup water
½ medium sweet potato, peeled and chopped
½ large head of broccoli, cut into florets
¼ white onion, diced
½ (15-ounce) can organic chickpeas, drained and rinsed
½ (28-ounce) can diced tomatoes
1 (14.5-ounce) can almond milk
2 tablespoons quinoa
1 garlic cloves, minced
1 tablespoon freshly grated ginger
1 tablespoon freshly grated turmeric
1 teaspoon wheat-free tamari sauce
½ teaspoon miso (or additional tamari)
¼ teaspoon chili flakes

Preparation
1. Combine all the ingredients in a slow cooker. Stir until everything is fully incorporated.
2. Turn the slow cooker to HIGH and cook for 3–4 hours, until sweet potato cooks through and the curry has thickened.

Nutrition facts per serving
Calories 507, total fat 32 g, carbs 50 g, protein 13 g, Sodium 380 mg, sugar 11 g

Salads And Sides

Slow-Cooked Mediterranean Zucchini Salad

The lively flavors of this Mediterranean zucchini salad make it an ideal companion to all dishes.

Serves 2 – Preparation time 15 minutes – Cooking time 8 hours

Ingredients
1 red onion, sliced
2 bell peppers, sliced
1 zucchini, sliced
1 (24-ounce) can whole tomatoes
1 tablespoon smoked paprika
2 teaspoons cumin
1 teaspoon salt
Fresh black pepper to taste
Juice of one lemon
Optional: falafel, to accompany

Preparation
1. Put the onion, bell peppers, zucchini, tomatoes, paprika, cumin, salt, black pepper and lemon juice in a large slow cooker, and cook on LOW for 7–8 hours.
2. After 8 hours, carefully open the lid, serve hot.
3. Falafel to go with it is also highly recommended.

Nutrition facts per serving
Calories 71.1, total fat 1.6 g, carbs 12.7 g, protein 3.5 g, Sodium 316.8 mg, sugar 0.5 g

German Potato Salad

Potato salad may never be the same after you make it in a slow cooker. Sun-dried tomatoes add flavor and texture to this summertime staple.

Serves 6 – Preparation time 20 minutes – Cooking time 7 hours

Ingredients
2 tablespoons olive oil
½ cup sun-dried tomato, chopped
1 cup onion, chopped
1 cup celery, chopped
1 teaspoon salt
½ teaspoon celery seed
¼ teaspoon black pepper
1 pound small red potatoes, sliced
1 cup vegetable broth
2 tablespoons sugar
1 tablespoon cornstarch
2 tablespoons cider vinegar
1 tablespoon chopped fresh parsley leaves

Preparation
1. Heat the oil in a medium skillet. Cook the sun-dried tomatoes until they begin to crisp up, and then set them aside. Add the onions and celery to the skillet, and cook until they begin to soften. Sprinkle with salt, celery seeds, and pepper.
2. Place half the potatoes in the slow cooker, and cover them with half the onion mixture. Repeat with the remaining potatoes and vegetables.
3. Pour the broth over the contents of the slow cooker.
4. Cover, and cook on LOW for 5–6 hours.
5. Remove the potatoes from the cooker with a skimmer. Mix the sugar, cornstarch, and vinegar in a small bowl, and pour the liquid in the cooker. Gently fold in the potatoes.
6. Increase the heat level to HIGH. Cover and cook for 20 to 30 minutes or until the sauce is warmed through, and the potatoes are tender. Transfer the salad to a serving bowl, and sprinkle with parsley leaves.

Nutrition facts per serving
Calories 280, total fat 5.5 g, carbs 12.7 g, protein 3.5 g, Sodium 316.8 mg, sugar 0.5 g

Garlic Cauliflower Mashed Potatoes

This dish is a game changer!

Serves 6 – Preparation time 15 minutes – Cooking time 4 hours

Ingredients
½ head of cauliflower
1 ½ cups water
2 large cloves garlic, peeled
½ teaspoon salt
1 bay leaf
½ tablespoon margarine
Salt and pepper to taste

Preparation
1. Cut the cauliflower into florets and place them in the slow cooker.
2. Add the water, garlic, salt, and bay leaf.
3. Cover, and cook on HIGH for 2–3 hours.
4. Remove the cloves of garlic and the bay leaf. Drain the water.
5. Add the margarine and let it melt.
6. Use a potato masher to make a cauliflower purée.
7. Season with salt and pepper to taste.

Nutrition facts per serving
Calories 96.4, total fat 5.9 g, carbs 10.4 g, protein 3.2 g, Sodium 553.7 mg, sugar 3.3 g

Farro Salad

Farro is an ancient grain that has a smooth texture and an earthy taste. This makes it an excellent base for hearty salads and side dishes.

Serves 4 – Preparation time 15 minutes – Cooking time 2 hours 10 minutes

Ingredients
1 cup uncooked faro
2 ¾ cups water
¼ cup cider vinegar
2 tablespoons canola oil
¼ teaspoon salt
¼ teaspoon ground black pepper
2 cups celery, finely chopped
1 cup parsley leaves, chopped
1 ¼ cups cherries, halved and pitted (can substitute grapes)

Preparation
1. In a slow cooker, combine the farro, water, and vinegar. Cover, and cook on HIGH for 2 hours.
2. **Remove the lid and let the farro cool for at least 10 – 15 minutes.**
3. In a medium bowl, combine the oil, salt, pepper, celery, and parsley. Stir in cooled farro to combine.
4. Add the cherries or grapes, stirring to combine. Serve.

Nutrition facts per serving

Calories 334, total fat 15 g, carbs 38 g, protein 13 g, Sodium 888 mg, sugar 5 g

Tofu And Black Bean Taco Salad

This simple blend of tofu, spices, garlic, and black beans makes a hearty taco filling. Pack the leftovers to put together the tacos for lunch.

Serves 4 – Preparation time 15 minutes – Cooking time 8 hours

Ingredients
1 ½ cups tofu, diced small
2 cups dried black beans
1 (18-ounce) can chili style diced tomatoes
2 tablespoons taco seasonings (like Old El Paso)
1 teaspoon cumin
1 tablespoon lime juice
1 clove garlic, minced
1 tablespoon molasses

For serving: Soft flour tortillas, lettuce, red onion, tomato, and cashew cream.

Preparation
1. Combine the tofu, beans, diced tomatoes, spices, and lime juice in the slow cooker. Cook on LOW for 6 – 8 hours, or until the beans are tender.

2. About 20–30 minutes before serving, turn the heat up to HIGH and lightly mash some of the beans and tofu, just enough to smash a few of the beans and thicken the filling. Stir in the garlic and the molasses. Replace the lid.
3. Serve with soft flour tortillas, lettuce, tomatoes, diced red onions, and your favourite taco toppings.

Nutrition facts per serving
Calories 218.9, total fat 1.3 g, carbs 28.2 g, protein 22.4 g,
Sodium 700 mg, sugar 6.3 g

Thai Summer Squash Salad With Peanut- Sauce

A flavorful, easy, and healthy cold "pasta" salad recipe! Easy to make ahead and feeds a crowd.

Serves 4 – Preparation time 15 minutes – Cooking time 8 hours

Ingredients
1 small spaghetti squash
2 cups water
2 cups broccoli, steamed
1 tablespoon sesame seeds
Optional toppings: chopped peanuts, sriracha

Light Thai Peanut Sauce
1 tablespoon brown sugar

2 tablespoons sesame oil
1 tablespoon rice wine vinegar
1 tablespoon soy sauce
2 tablespoons peanut butter
1 teaspoon ginger root, peeled and grated
1 clove garlic, minced
¼ teaspoon salt
Pinch red pepper flakes
½ teaspoon sriracha (optional)

Preparation
1. Pierce your spaghetti squash with a fork.
2. Place the spaghetti squash and 2 cups of water in a slow cooker. Close the lid and cook for 8–9 hours on LOW.
3. When done, remove the spaghetti squash from the slow cooker and let it cool for 20–30 minutes. Discard the water.
4. While the squash is cooling, prepare the sauce by combining all the ingredients in a small bowl.
5. After the squash has cooled, cut it in half and scoop out the seeds and pulp.
6. With the pulp removed, use a fork to shred the insides of the squash into spaghetti-like noodles.
7. Divide the "noodles" among four serving bowls and top each with ½ cup of broccoli, 3 tablespoons of dressing, a generous pinch of sesame seeds, and peanuts if desired. Enjoy!

Nutrition facts per serving

Calories 145.9, total fat 4.3 g, carbs 26.2 g, protein 5.4 g,
Sodium 108 mg, sugar 8.3 g

Stews And Chilis

Vegan Four Bean Chili

This slow cooker vegetarian chili is vegan, gluten free, SO healthy, and loaded with veggies, spices, and different kinds of beans.

Serves 4– Preparation time 20 minutes – Cooking time 6 hours

Ingredients
1 tablespoon olive oil
1 large onion, chopped
1 green bell pepper, chopped
1 zucchini, chopped
2 stalks celery, chopped
3 garlic cloves, chopped
1 (11-ounce) can condensed black bean soup (or canned black beans in juice)
1 (15-ounce) can kidney beans, drained and rinsed
1 (15-ounce) can chickpeas, drained and rinsed (may substitute lentils)
1 (16-ounce) can vegetarian baked beans

1 (14.5-ounce) can chopped tomato puree (or a 28-ounce can of crushed tomatoes)
1 (15-ounce) can whole kernel corn, drained
1 (4-ounce) can diced chilies
1 jalapeño pepper, chopped (reduce the amount for milder chili)
1 tablespoon chili powder
1 teaspoon cumin
1 tablespoon dried parsley
1 tablespoon dried oregano
1 tablespoon dried basil
1 teaspoon marjoram

Preparation
1. Heat the olive oil in a medium skillet. Sauté the onion, pepper, zucchini and celery in a pan for about 5 minutes. Add the garlic, and cook until fragrant.
2. In a slow cooker, mix the black bean soup, kidney beans, chickpeas, baked beans, tomatoes, corn, chilies, jalapeño, and the vegetable mixture.
3. Season with the chili powder, cumin, parsley, oregano, basil, and marjoram.
4. Cook for about 6 hours on LOW.
5. Serve with tortillas, vegan cornbread, rice, or French bread.

Nutrition facts per serving

Calories 263, total fat 2.3 g, carbs 51.9 g, protein 12.9 g,
Sodium 240 mg, sugar 4.6

Mushroom Lentil Buckwheat Stew

These flavors combine very well to give you a healthy, earthy taste. Serve with garlic bread.

Serves 4 – Preparation time 15 minutes – Cooking time 12 hours

Ingredients
4 cups vegetable broth
1 cup sliced fresh button mushrooms
½ ounce dried shiitake mushrooms, torn into pieces
¼ cup uncooked buckwheat
¼ cup dry lentils
2 tablespoons dried onion flakes
1 teaspoon garlic, minced
1 teaspoon dried summer savory
2 bay leaves
½ teaspoon dried basil
1 teaspoon ground black pepper
Salt to taste

Preparation
1. In a slow cooker, combine all the ingredients.
2. Cover, and cook for 10–12 hours on LOW. Remove the bay leaves before serving.

Nutrition facts per serving
Calories 224, total fat 7.5 g, carbs 32.5 g, protein 5.6 g, Sodium 1240 mg, sugar 5.1

Corn And Red Pepper Chowder

Cozy up to a bowl of this creamy potato, corn, and red pepper chowder that's ready in few hours.

Serves 4 – Preparation time 15 minutes – Cooking time 10 hours

Ingredients
1 tablespoon olive oil
½ medium yellow onion, diced
½ medium red bell pepper, seeded and diced
2 medium red-skinned potatoes, diced
2 cups frozen sweet corn kernels, divided
2 cups vegetable broth
½ teaspoon ground cumin
¼ teaspoon smoked paprika
Pinch cayenne pepper
½ teaspoon kosher salt
½ cup coconut milk
 Salt and black pepper to taste
 To garnish: chopped red bell pepper, corn kernels, and sliced scallions

Preparation

1. Heat the olive oil in a medium-sized pan over medium heat. Add the onion and cook, stirring occasionally, until light and smooth, about 5 minutes. Transfer the onion, along with the red pepper, potatoes, 1 cup of corn, broth, cumin, smoked paprika, cayenne pepper, and salt to the slow cooker.
2. Cook on LOW for 8–10 hours, until the potatoes are tender.
3. Turn off the slow cooker and remove the lid. Let the soup cool down a bit. Blend the soup with a hand blender or a standard blender. Put it back in the pot and turn it back on.
4. Add the remaining 1 cup of corn, and the coconut milk. Cover, and heat on HIGH for 20–30 minutes, until it is warmed through. Season with salt and pepper.
5. Serve with additional corn, peppers and/or sliced green onions.

Nutrition facts per serving
Calories 85, total fat 2.2 g, carbs 16.2 g, protein 2.6 g, Sodium 163 mg, sugar 3.4

Lentil Chili

This thick and rich vegan chili is different enough to be special, but it still has a fairly popular taste to please most people. It's the perfect chili for the fall!

Serves 4 – Preparation time 10 minutes – Cooking time 8 hours

Ingredients
½ medium onion, diced
2 cloves garlic, minced
½ jalapeño, diced, seeds removed
½ red pepper, chopped
½ yellow pepper, chopped
½ large carrot, peeled and diced
1 ½ cups vegetable broth
1 (15-ounce) can tomato sauce
1 (15-ounce) can diced tomatoes
8 ounces brown lentils, rinsed
1 (15-ounce) cans small red kidney beans, rinsed and drained
2 tablespoons chili powder
½ tablespoon cumin
Salt and black pepper, to taste

Preparation
1. Place the onion, garlic, jalapeño, red pepper, yellow pepper, carrot, vegetable broth, tomato sauce, diced tomatoes, brown lentils, red beans, chili powder, cumin, and salt and black pepper in a slow cooker. Stir well to combine.
2. Cover and cook on LOW for 6 hours. Serve warm.

Nutrition facts per serving

Calories 285, total fat 2 g, carbs 50.6 g, protein 19.1 g, Sodium 671 mg, sugar 7.4

Black Bean And Quinoa Crock-Pot Stew

It's hearty, easy to make, and tastes amazing. This stew is vegan and gluten free.

Serves 4 – Preparation time 10 minutes – Cooking time 10 hours

Ingredients
1 dried chipotle pepper
8 ounces dried organic black beans, rinsed and cleaned
¼ cup uncooked quinoa, rinsed and cleaned
½ (28-ounce) can organic diced tomatoes
½ red onion, diced
2 cloves garlic, minced
½ green bell pepper, chopped
½ red bell pepper, chopped
½ dried cinnamon stick
1 teaspoon chili powder
½ teaspoon ground coriander
2 tablespoons fresh cilantro, chopped
3 ½ cups water
Salt and pepper to taste

Toppings
Cilantro
Green onions, thinly sliced
Lime wedges
Avocado
Tortilla chips

Preparation
1. Combine all the ingredients EXCEPT the salt in the slow cooker, and stir.
2. Cook on HIGH for 4–6 hours, or on LOW for 8–10 hours, until the black beans are tender.
3. Taste the mixture, and add salt as needed. Remove the chipotle pepper before serving.
4. Serve topped with fresh cilantro, green onions, a squeeze of fresh lime juice, diced avocados, tortilla chips, etc.

Nutrition facts per serving
Calories 310, total fat 2.5 g, carbs 576 g, protein 17 g, Sodium 150 mg, sugar 5.4

Lentil Cauliflower Stew

An easy slow cooker recipe for cauliflower stew with lentils for a healthful, stick-to-your-ribs meal.

Serves 6 – Preparation time 30 minutes – Cooking time 8 hours

Ingredients
1 tablespoon olive oil
2 onions, chopped
2 cloves garlic, chopped
16 ounces dried lentils
1 large head cauliflower, chopped into very small florets
2 leeks (white and green parts only) halved, washed carefully, and chopped
2 large carrots, peeled and chopped
3 celery ribs, chopped
2 bay leaves
1 tablespoon fresh thyme or 1 teaspoon dried thyme
2 tablespoons kosher salt (or to taste)
1 teaspoon cumin
½ teaspoon cayenne
¼ teaspoon black pepper
8 cups low sodium vegetable broth
32 ounces canned tomatoes with juice, diced
2 cups kale, chopped

For topping, optional: cashew cream, chopped coriander or parsley, green onion

Preparation
1. Heat the oil in a saucepan over medium heat. Cook the onions for about 4 minutes, until soft. Add the chopped garlic and sauté for another minute.

2. Pour the onions and garlic into the slow cooker, and add the remaining ingredients.
3. Cover the slow cooker and cook on HIGH for 6 hours, or for 8 hours on LOW.
4. Remove the bay leaves before serving.
5. Serve hot with your choice of toppings.

Nutrition facts per serving
Calories 160, total fat 6 g, carbs 19 g, protein 7 g, Sodium 690 mg, sugar 10 g

Root Vegetable And Tempeh Vegan Chili

This chili recipe packs a powerful protein boost and has a satisfying texture. It's also gluten free.

Serves 6 – Preparation time 10 minutes – Cooking time 6 hours

Ingredients
1 cup rutabaga, peeled and cubed
1 cup turnip, peeled and cubed
1 cup sweet potato, peeled and cubed
1 cup parsnip, peeled and cubed
½ cup carrots, peeled and cubed
½ cup beets, peeled and cubed
½ cup yellow onion, diced
4 ounces gluten-free tempeh, rinsed and cubed
½ cup vegetable broth

½ (28-ounce) can diced tomatoes
½ (15-ounce) can kidney beans, rinsed
½ (15-ounce) can black beans, rinsed
½ teaspoon kosher sea salt, divided
½ teaspoon cayenne pepper, divided
½ teaspoon chili powder, divided
½ teaspoon ground cumin, divided
¼ teaspoon paprika, divided
¼ teaspoon nutmeg, divided

Toppings:
½ cup vegan sour cream, for garnish
½ cup vegan cheese shreds, for garnish
¼ cup flat leaf parsley, chopped, for garnish

Preparation
1. Peel and cut the vegetables into ½-inch cubes, keeping all the pieces the same size so they cook evenly. Mix the vegetables together in a 6-quart slow cooker.
2. Rinse and cut the tempeh into ½-inch cubes, then layer it over the vegetables.
3. Pour the vegetable stock and the diced tomatoes over the tempeh, and add the kidney and black beans.
4. Cover the slow cooker and set it on LOW. After 2 hours, add the spices and stir to combine all the ingredients. Put the lid back on and cook for another 4 hours.

5. After a total of six hours, check the stew. If the vegetables and the tempeh are soft, turn off the slow cooker and serve the chili. Otherwise, cook for another hour on LOW.
6. Serve the chili in large bowls with toppings.

Nutrition facts per serving
Calories 260, total fat 7.1 g, carbs 35.8 g, protein 17.3 g,
Sodium 822.2 mg, sugar 8.1g

Vegetable Recipes

Balsamic Pear, Mushroom, And Asparagus

An unusual blend of spices enlivens this slow-cooked dish, which benefits from the abundance of asparagus in the spring. In other seasons, fresh green beans would be a good option to replace asparagus.

Serves 4 – Preparation time 10 minutes – Cooking time 6 hours

Ingredients
1 tablespoon vegetable oil
2 pounds mushrooms, sliced
1 onion, sliced
2 ripe Bartlett pears, cored and sliced
1 pound fresh asparagus, trimmed

4 cloves garlic, minced
2 tablespoons balsamic vinegar
3 tablespoons apple juice
1 teaspoon dried rosemary
1 tablespoon fresh ginger, grated
2 tablespoons dark brown sugar
Salt and pepper

Preparation
1. Heat the oil in a saucepan over medium heat. Cook the mushrooms in the hot oil until golden, 3–5 minutes. Transfer them to a slow cooker.
2. Add the onion to the mushrooms, and season with salt and pepper. Add the pears and asparagus.
3. In a medium-sized bowl, combine the garlic, balsamic vinegar, apple juice, rosemary, ginger, and sugar in a bowl; pour it over the asparagus. Season with salt and pepper.
4. Cook over LOW for 4 to 6 hours.

Nutrition facts per serving
Calories 255, total fat 3 g, carbs 27.8 g, protein 27.6 g, Sodium 214.2 mg, sugar 8.1g

Baked Sweet Potatoes

Cooking sweet potatoes in the slow cooker makes them extra moist and sweet!

Serves 4 – Preparation time 10 minutes – Cooking time 8 hours

Ingredients
4 medium sweet potatoes, washed and dried
4 sheets of aluminum foil

Preparation
1. Poke the sweet potatoes 3–4 times with a fork.
2. Wrap each sweet potato in aluminum foil and place them in the slow cooker, and cover. You do not need any liquid in the slow cooker.
3. Cook on LOW for 8 hours, or until tender.

Nutrition facts per serving
Calories 316, total fat 3.4 g, carbs 29.3 g, protein 41.2 g,
Sodium 1561.3 mg, sugar 3.1 g

Enchilada Amaranth

This easy slow cooker recipe is a family favorite! Serve tortilla chips or tortillas on the side!

Serves 4 – Preparation time 15 minutes – Cooking time 6 hours

Ingredients
1 cup uncooked amaranth, rinsed

½ cup water
1 small onion, diced
2 cloves garlic, minced
1 red pepper, seeds removed, diced
2 (15-ounce) cans black beans, rinsed and drained
2 (10-ounce) cans red enchilada sauce
1 (15-ounce) can diced tomatoes
1 (4.5-ounce) can chopped green chilies
1 cup corn frozen kernels
Juice of 1 small lime
1 teaspoon ground cumin
1 tablespoon chili powder
⅓ cup chopped cilantro
Salt and black pepper, to taste
1 ½ cups shredded vegan cheese

Optional toppings: Sliced green onions, avocado, diced tomatoes, cashew cream, cilantro, and lime wedges

Preparation
1. Mix the all the ingredients EXCEPT the cheese in a 6-quart slow cooker. Mix to combine. Season with salt and pepper. Cover, and cook on HIGH for 3 hours, or on LOW 6 hours, until the amaranth is cooked.
2. Remove the lid and mix the casserole. Test and adjust the spice if necessary. Stir in half the cheese, and sprinkle the other half on top. Replace the lid, and cook until the cheese has melted, about 15 minutes.
3. Serve hot with the desired toppings.

Nutrition facts per serving
Calories 270, total fat 9.7 g, carbs 38.1 g, protein 11.6 g,
Sodium 468.3 mg, sugar 4.5 g

Rosemary And Red Pepper Tofu

Lunch won't be dull with this tasty, make-ahead meal.

Serves 4 – Preparation time 20 minutes – Cooking time 6 hours

Ingredients
1 small onion, thinly sliced
1 medium red bell pepper, seeded and thinly sliced
4 cloves garlic, minced
2 teaspoons dried rosemary
½ teaspoon dried oregano
8s tofu
¼ teaspoon coarsely ground pepper
¼ cup dry vermouth
1 ½ tablespoons cornstarch
2 tablespoons cold water
Salt to taste
¼ cup chopped fresh parsley

Preparation
1. In a 6-quart slow cooker, combine the onion, bell pepper, garlic, rosemary, and oregano. Add the

tofu, and arrange it in a single layer over the onion. Sprinkle with pepper. Pour in the vermouth. Cover, and cook on LOW for 5–7 hours.
2. Transfer tofu to a warm, deep platter, and cover to keep warm.
3. In a small bowl, stir together the cornstarch and cold water. Stir it
4. into the cooking liquid in the slow cooker. Increase the heat to HIGH, and cover. Cook, stirring a few times, until sauce is thickened (about 10 more minutes).
5. Season to taste with salt. Spoon the sauce over the tofu, and sprinkle with parsley.

Nutrition facts per serving
Calories 165, total fat 1.6 g, carbs 3.5 g, protein 27.8 g, Sodium 226.3 mg, sugar 0.9 g

Quick And Easy Swiss Cauliflower

Need healthy slow cooker recipes? We've got you covered! This veggie-filled side dish will go great with just about any meal.

Serves 6– Preparation time 25 minutes – Cooking time 6 hours

Ingredients
2 cups broccoli florets
2 cups cauliflower florets

½ (14-ounce) jar vegan alfredo pasta sauce
3 ounces vegan Swiss cheese, sliced
½ large onion, chopped
½ teaspoon dried thyme, oregano, or basil, crushed
⅛ teaspoon ground black pepper
¼ cup sliced almonds

Preparation
1. In a 4-quart slow cooker, combine the broccoli, cauliflower, pasta sauce, vegan cheese, onion, thyme, and pepper.
2. Cover, and cook on LOW for 6–7 hours, or on HIGH for 3 hours.
3. Stir gently before serving. If desired, sprinkle with almonds.

Nutrition facts per serving
Calories 177, total fat 12 g, carbs 10 g, protein 27.8 g, Sodium 573 mg sugar 4g

Tempeh With Apples, Sweet Potatoes, And Sauerkraut

In this lovely side, sweet potatoes are slow-cooked with apples and spices. It's perfect for any special occasion.

 Serves 4 – Preparation time 15 minutes – Cooking time 5hours

Ingredients
2 large apples, peeled, cored, and cut into bite-sized pieces
4 medium sweet potatoes, peeled and cut into 1 ½-inch pieces
1 ½ cups apple juice or ¾ cup apple cider
20 ounces tempeh
4 cups wine-cured sauerkraut
1 teaspoon caraway seed (optional)
⅔ cup honey mustard

Preparation
1. Arrange the apple and sweet potato in the bottom of the slow cooker. Pour in the apple juice.
2. Add the tempeh, and cover it with the sauerkraut. Sprinkle in the caraway seed.
3. Smear the mustard on top.
4. Cover, and cook on LOW for 5 hours.

Nutrition facts per serving
Calories 120, total fat 2.9 g, carbs 24.7 g, protein 0.8 g, Sodium 15.3 mg, sugar 4 g

Vegetable Red Curry

This is a satisfying and comforting vegan dish packed with protein and full of flavor, thanks to the warm spices.

Serves 6 – Preparation time 15 minutes – Cooking time 7 hours

Ingredients
4 tablespoons red curry paste
2 cups full fat coconut milk
1 tablespoon creamy peanut butter
4 cups vegetable broth
2 tablespoons maple syrup
8 scallions, chopped
2 red bell peppers, sliced into strips
2 green bell peppers, sliced into strips
4 cups chickpeas
2 cups carrots, sliced
2 tablespoons ginger, freshly minced
2 tablespoons soy sauce
2 Thai chilies, thinly sliced
2 tablespoons fresh lime juice
1 cup rice
⅓ cup Thai basil

Preparation
1. Stir the red curry paste with the coconut milk and peanut butter until smooth. Spoon the mixture into the slow cooker, and add the broth, maple syrup, scallions, red bell pepper, green bell pepper, chickpeas, carrots, ginger, soy sauce, Thai chilies, and lime juice.
2. Cover, and cook on LOW for 6 hours.

3. Add the rice. Increase the heat to HIGH and cook for 30–45 minutes, depending on the type of rice.
4. Add the Thai basil, and serve immediately.

Nutrition facts per serving
Calories 164, total fat 7.6 g, carbs 17.3 g, protein 7.2 g, Sodium 449.6 mg, sugar 3.3 g

Mediterranean Stuffed Peppers

Hearty peppers loaded with protein and fiber, and packed with so much flavor, all made in the slow cooker.

Serves 2 – Preparation time 15 minutes – Cooking time 4 hours

Ingredients
2 large bell peppers
½ (15-ounce) can cannellini beans, rinsed and drained
¼ cup couscous, cooked
2 scallions, white and green parts separated, thinly sliced
1 clove garlic, minced
½ teaspoon dried oregano
Coarse salt and freshly ground pepper
Lemon wedges, for serving

Preparation

1. Cut a very thin layer off the base of each pepper so they sit flat. Slice the top, straight across under the stem, to make a cup. Discard the stems. Remove the ribs and seeds from the peppers.
2. Add the beans, couscous, scallions (the white parts), garlic, and oregano to the bowl. Season with salt and pepper, and mix. Fill the peppers with the bean mixture, and place them in the slow cooker in a vertical position. Cover, and cook on HIGH for 4 hours.
3. Sprinkle the peppers with the scallion greens, and serve with lemon slices.

Nutrition facts per serving
Calories 380, total fat 22.3 g, carbs 27.3 g, protein 17.2 g,
Sodium 222 mg, sugar 1.3 g

Summer Vegetable Succotash Recipe

The word **succotash** comes from a Narragansett word, which means cooked corn. The dish is a soothing combination of corn, beans, and other local, seasonal vegetables.

Serves 4 – Preparation time 15 minutes – Cooking time 4 hours

Ingredients
½ (10-ounce) can seasoned diced tomatoes in juice

¼ cup vegetable broth
1 cup corn kernels
1 cup diced zucchini
½ cup sliced okra
3 tablespoons white onion, minced
2 cloves garlic, minced
¼ teaspoon salt
⅛ teaspoon ground black pepper
⅛ teaspoon red pepper flakes
1 tablespoon lemon juice
¼ teaspoon hot sauce
¼ teaspoon dried parsley

Preparation
1. Put the slow cooker on LOW. Add the tomatoes with their juice, and the vegetable broth.
2. Add the corn, zucchini, okra, onion, and garlic. Sprinkle with the salt, pepper, and red pepper flakes. Mix to combine.
3. Cover, and cook for 4 hours on LOW.
4. Before serving the succotash, mix the lemon juice and the hot sauce. Add the parsley and mix.
5. Spoon the mixture over the succotash, and stir to combine.

Nutrition facts per serving
Calories 206, total fat 10.8 g, carbs 27.3 g, protein 4.4 g,
Sodium 197.2 mg, sugar 9.4 g

Eggplant Lasagna

Healthy, gluten free, and your slow cooker does all the work! Slow cooker Low Carb Lasagna is made with eggplant in place of pasta.

Serves 6 – Preparation time 20 minutes – Cooking time 4 hours

Ingredients
1 medium eggplant (1 pound), cut into ¼-inch thick rounds
2 teaspoons salt
1 container soft (silken) tofu
1 container firm or extra firm tofu
¼ cup soy milk
2 cups vegan ricotta
2 tablespoons chopped fresh basil
2 cloves garlic, minced
1 teaspoon Italian seasoning
3 ½ cups marinara sauce, warmed
1 cup vegan cheese blend

Preparation
1. Arrange the eggplant in a single layer on 2 racks. Sprinkle with 1 teaspoon salt. Let stand for 10 minutes. Turn the slices and repeat the process. Rinse off the salt, and dry the slices between clean kitchen towels.

2. In a food processor or blender, combine the silken tofu, the firm or extra-firm tofu, and the soy milk.
3. Combine the vegan ricotta with the tofu mixture, and add the basil, garlic, and Italian seasoning in a bowl.
4. Coat a slow cooker with cooking spray. Add ¾ cup warm marinara sauce. Top with eggplant slices, overlapping to fit. Spread half of the ricotta mixture over the eggplant. Layer on more eggplant slices, and then 1 cup of the marinara sauce and ¼ cup shredded vegan cheese. Repeat with another layer of eggplant, remaining ricotta mixture, remaining eggplant, 1 cup marinara sauce and ¼ cup shredded cheese. Finish with the last of the marinara, reserving ½ cup of the shredded cheese for later.
5. Cover, and cook 4–5 hours on low. Sprinkle the remaining ½ cup vegan cheese over the top. Cover, and let it stand until the cheese melts. Uncover, and cool for 20 minutes.
6. Serve and enjoy!

Nutrition facts per serving
Calories 420, total fat 18.9 g, carbs 37.1 g, protein 36.1 g,
Sodium 1500 mg, sugar 8.2 g

Soups And Bowls

Yellow Pea Soup

Something magical happens when the split peas break down into a thick soup, naturally creamy and delicious after several hours in the slow cooker.

Serves 4 – Preparation time 10 minutes – Cooking time 8 hours

Ingredients
1 pound yellow split peas, rinsed and sorted
1 cup carrots, julienned
½ teaspoon dried thyme leaves
½ teaspoon dried marjoram leaves
¼ teaspoon pepper
2 cups vegetable broth
1 ½ cups water

Preparation
1. In 3- to 4-quart slow cooker, mix the yellow split peas, carrots, thyme, marjoram, pepper, vegetable broth, and water.
2. Cover, and cook on LOW for 8–10 hours.
3. Increase the heat setting to HIGH, and stir well. Cover and cook 30 minutes longer.

Nutrition facts per serving
Calories 198, total fat 4.7 g, carbs 21.3g, protein 18.2 g, Sodium 1466.5 mg, sugar 3.6 g

Lentil Tortilla Soup

This easy and crazy flavorful soup can be made in a pressure cooker or a slow cooker.

Serves 4 – Preparation time 10 minutes – Cooking time 6 hours

Ingredients
1 cup onion, diced
1 teaspoon avocado oil or olive oil
1 bell pepper, diced
1 jalapeño pepper, diced
2 ½ cups vegetable broth
1 (15-ounce) can tomato sauce or crushed tomatoes, extra to taste
½ cup salsa verde (or your favorite salsa!)
1 tablespoon tomato paste
1 (15-ounce) can black beans, drained and rinsed
1 (15-ounce) can pinto beans, drained and rinsed
1 cup corn (fresh, canned, or frozen)
¾ cup dried red lentils
½ teaspoon chili powder
½ teaspoon garlic powder
½ teaspoon cumin
¼ teaspoon cayenne pepper
¼-½ cup cashew cream
Salt and pepper to taste
Toppings of your choice

Preparation

1. In a 6-quart slow cooker, combine all the ingredients EXCEPT the cream and toppings. Cook on HIGH for 5–6 hours, until the lentils are cooked through and the veggies are tender.
2. Swirl in the cashew cream, add all your favourite toppings, and serve.

Nutrition facts per serving
Calories 188, total fat 5.6g, carbs 25 g, protein 11.6 g, Sodium 369.5 mg, sugar 4.4 g

Lemon Rosemary Lentil Soup

Fresh vegetables, lemon, and rosemary become an amazingly hearty soup with minimal effort.

Serves 4 – Preparation time 15 minutes – Cooking time 6 hours

Ingredients
3 carrots, peeled and diced
½ large onion, diced
2 cloves garlic, minced
½ yellow pepper, chopped
Pinch cayenne pepper
1 ½ cups red lentils
2 cups vegetable broth

1 ½ cups water
1 teaspoon salt
½ teaspoon lemon zest
Juice of half a lemon
½ tablespoon fresh rosemary, chopped, plus some for garnish

Preparation
1. In a 6-quart slow cooker, combine the carrots, onion, garlic, yellow pepper, cayenne pepper, red lentils, broth, water, and salt.
2. Cook on LOW for 6 hours.
3. Add the lemon zest, juice, and rosemary. Season with salt and pepper.
4. Pour into bowls and garnish with extra chopped rosemary.

Nutrition facts per serving
Calories 410, total fat 25g, carbs 69 g, protein 29 g, Sodium 680 mg, sugar 6 g

Lentil And Potato Soup

Warm, comforting lentil soup can be in your belly in couple of hours.

Serves 4 – Preparation time 20minutes – Cooking time 8 hours

Ingredients

½ tablespoon olive oil
½ large yellow onion, chopped
½ celery stalk, sliced
½ large carrot, sliced
1 clove garlic, minced
½ large bunch Swiss chard, leaves torn into bite-sized pieces and stems sliced
½ cup dried brown lentils, picked over and rinsed
2 medium potatoes, cut into 1-inch pieces
3 cups vegetable broth
½ tablespoon soy sauce or tamari
Salt and pepper to taste

Preparation

1. Heat the oil in a large pan over medium heat. Add the onion, celery, carrot, garlic, and chard stalks. Cover and cook until tender, about 8–10 minutes, stirring occasionally.
2. Put the cooked vegetable mixture, lentils, potatoes, broth, and soy sauce in a 4- to 6-quart slow cooker. Stir to combine, cover, and cook on LOW for 8 hours.
3. Just before the soup is ready, boil a large pot of water. Put the reserved chard leaves in the boiling water and simmer for about 5 minutes. Drain well and stir them into the soup. Season with salt and pepper.

Nutrition facts per serving

Calories 175.3 total fat 5.1g, carbs 27 g, protein 9.6 g, Sodium 396.1 mg, sugar 3.6 g

Butternut Squash And Parsnip Soup

This delicious butternut squash and parsnip soup will warm you up on a cold winter's night. Serve with fresh bread and a salad for a complete meal.

Serves 4 – Preparation time 20 minutes – Cooking time 8 hours

Ingredients
2 ½ cups butternut squash, peeled, seeded, and chopped
1 cup parsnips, peeled and chopped
1 cup onion, chopped
½ cup apple, peeled and chopped
1 cup vegetable broth
½ teaspoon salt
¼ teaspoon black pepper
¼ teaspoon dried thyme
⅛ teaspoon paprika
¼ cup soy or almond milk

Preparation

1. Combine all the ingredients EXCEPT the milk in a slow cooker. Cook on LOW for 6 hours, or HIGH for 3–4 hours
2. Once the vegetables are soft, purée the soup in a blender in until smooth.
3. Return the soup to the slow cooker and stir in the milk.

Nutrition facts per serving
Calories 238 total fat 9.2 g, carbs 35.3 g, protein 6 g, Sodium 199 mg, sugar 9.9 g

Desserts

Caramel Poached Peaches

This easy dessert is bursting with juicy apples, brown sugar, and an oat crumble topping.

Serves 4 – Preparation time 10 minutes – Cooking time 4 hours

Ingredients
For the peaches:
1 cup brown sugar
½ cup granulated sugar
5 large peaches, peeled and cut into chunks
¼ teaspoon salt
1 teaspoon cinnamon

For the topping:
⅔ cup oats
⅔ cup loosely packed brown sugar
¼ cup flour
½ teaspoon cinnamon
3–4 tablespoons soft margarine
1 teaspoon vanilla extract

Preparation
1. Mix the brown sugar, granulated sugar, apples, salt, and cinnamon in a mixing bowl. Layer the mixture on the bottom of the slow cooker.
2. Combine the oats, brown sugar, flour, cinnamon, margarine, and vanilla extract. Sprinkle the mixture over the apples. Cook on LOW for 4 hours.
3. Turn off the heat and let it sit for an hour, to thicken the caramel.

Nutrition facts per serving
Calories 275 total fat 3.4 g, carbs 82.7 g, protein 0 g, Sodium 32.1 mg, sugar 76.5 g

Lemon Blueberry Cake

This blueberry lemon cake recipe is perfect for spring.

Serves 4 – Preparation time 10 minutes – Cooking time 1 hour

Ingredients
½ cup whole wheat pastry flour
¼ teaspoon stevia, or to taste
¼ teaspoon baking powder
⅓ cup unsweetened non-dairy milk
¼ cup blueberries
1 teaspoon ground flax seed mixed with 2 teaspoons warm water
1 teaspoon olive oil
½ teaspoon lemon zest
¼ teaspoon vanilla extract
¼ teaspoon lemon extract

Preparation
1. Spray the slow cooker with oil.
2. Combine the flour, stevia, and baking powder in a medium bowl.
3. In a separate bowl, mix the non-dairy milk, blueberries, flax seed with water, olive oil, lemon zest, vanilla extract, and lemon extract.
4. Add the wet ingredients to the dry, and mix until combined.
5. Pour the mixture into the slow cooker and spread it evenly on the bottom.
6. Put a clean dish towel or paper towel between the lid and slow cooker to absorb the condensation. Cook on HIGH for 1 hour, or until the middle is firm.

Nutrition facts per serving
Calories 182.5, total fat 2.3 g, carbs 37.4 g, protein 4.0 g,
Sodium 390 mg, sugar 15 g

Caramel Mocha Cheesecake

It is hard to believe that you can cook a cheesecake...a VEGAN CHEESECAKE in your crock pot, but you sure can.

Serves 4– Preparation time 10 minutes – Cooking time 4 hours

Ingredients
Mocha cheesecake:
¾ cup ground vegan chocolate graham crackers or chocolate wafers (such as chocolate chip Teddy Grahams®)
4 tablespoons margarine, melted
⅓ cup sugar
8 ounces vegan cream cheese, softened
1 banana
1 ounce bittersweet vegan chocolate, melted and slightly cooled
½ teaspoon pure vanilla extract
½ teaspoon instant coffee
⅛ teaspoon salt

Salted caramel:

4 tablespoons margarine
1 cup brown sugar, packed
½ cup almond milk
½ teaspoon sea salt or Kosher salt
1 tablespoon pure vanilla extract
Cashew cream for serving (optional)

Preparation
1. Coat six 4-ounce ramekins with a non-stick spray.
2. Mix the crushed grahams with the margarine and a pinch of salt. In each ramekin, put a tablespoon and a teaspoon of the crust mixture. Press the crust into a uniform layer.
3. Beat the sugar and vegan cream cheese in a large bowl until smooth. Add the banana and mix until combined. Mix in the melted chocolate, vanilla, instant coffee, and salt. Pour the filling into each ramekin up to ¾ of its capacity and place it in the slow cooker.
4. Carefully pour warm water around the ramekins until three-quarters is submerged. Cover and cook for 1 ½ hours on HIGH.
5. When the cheesecakes are set, carefully remove them from the slow cooker and refrigerate for 2 hours.
6. To make the salted caramel, combine the margarine, brown sugar, almond milk, and salt in a medium saucepan. Cook for 7 minutes over medium heat, stirring occasionally. Add the vanilla and cook

for 1 more minute to thicken. Pour the caramel into a mason jar, and refrigerate until it is cold.
7. Spoon salted caramel sauce and cashew cream over each cheesecake just before serving.

Nutrition facts per serving
Calories 370, total fat 14 g, carbs 53 g, protein 10 g, Sodium 290 mg sugar 46.5 g

Triple Chocolate-Peanut Butter Pudding Cake

This delicious recipe for slow cooked cake will satisfy all cravings. Three kinds of chocolate give this slow-cooked cake its characteristic chocolate flavor.

Serves 4 – Preparation time 20 minutes – Cooking time 2 hours

Ingredients
Nonstick cooking spray
1 cup all-purpose flour
⅓ cup sugar
2 tablespoons unsweetened cocoa powder
1 ½ teaspoons baking powder
½ cup chocolate almond milk
2 tablespoons vegetable oil
2 teaspoons vanilla
½ cup vegan peanut butter-flavored baking chips

½ cup chocolate pieces
½ cup chopped peanuts
¾ cup sugar
2 tablespoons unsweetened cocoa powder
1 ½ cups boiling water
Vegan chocolate pieces (optional, to garnish)

Preparation
1. Lightly coat the inside of a 4-quart slow cooker with cooking spray, or line the bowl with parchment paper.
2. In a medium bowl, mix the flour, sugar, cocoa powder, and baking powder. Add the chocolate almond milk, oil, and vanilla. Stir just until moistened.
3. Stir in the peanut butter baking ships, the chocolate pieces, and peanuts.
4. Spread the mixture in the slow cooker.
5. In another medium bowl, mix ¾ cup sugar and 2 tablespoons cocoa powder. Slowly add the boiling water. Carefully pour the hot cocoa mixture onto the mixture in the slow cooker.
6. Cover, and cook on HIGH for 2–2 ½ hours, or until a toothpick inserted in the center of the cake comes out clean.
7. Remove the liner from the bowl, if possible, or turn off the pot. Let the cake rest for 30–40 minutes, to cool slightly.
8. To serve, spoon the cake onto serving dishes and garnish with chocolate pieces.

Nutrition facts per serving
Calories 276.5, total fat 13.7 g, carbs 29.3 g, protein 5.1 g,
Sodium 357 mg, sugar 10.6 g

Apple Crisp

An easy way to make a wonderful, comforting meal with these abundantly falling apples!

Serves 6– Preparation time 30 minutes – Cooking time 3 hours

Ingredients
1 cup all-purpose flour
½ cup light brown sugar
½ cup white sugar
½ teaspoon ground cinnamon
¼ teaspoon ground nutmeg
1 pinch salt
½ cup margarine
1 cup chopped walnuts
⅓ cup white sugar, or to taste
1 tablespoon cornstarch
½ teaspoon ground ginger
½ teaspoon ground cinnamon
6 cups apples, peeled, cored, and chopped
2 tablespoons lemon juice

Preparation
1. Mix the flour, brown sugar, ½ cup white sugar, ½ teaspoon cinnamon, nutmeg, and salt in a bowl. Combine the margarine with the flour mixture, using your fingers or a fork, until coarse crumbs form. Stir in the nuts and set the bowl aside.
2. Whisk together ⅓ cup of sugar, cornstarch, ginger, and ½ teaspoon of cinnamon.
3. Put the apples in a slow cooker, and incorporate the cornstarch mixture. Mix in the lemon juice.
4. Sprinkle the crumble mixture on top. Cover and cook for 2 hours on HIGH, or 4 hours on LOW, until the apples are soft.
5. Let the dish cool for an hour before serving.

Nutrition facts per serving
Calories 187, total fat 7.7 g, carbs 30.2 g, protein 1.5 g, Sodium 147.6 mg, sugar 12 g

Turmeric Rice Pudding

Fragrant, rich, and deliciously creamy.

Serves 2 – Preparation time 10 minutes – Cooking time 6 hours

Ingredients
½ cup rice
1 ½ cups almond milk

1 teaspoon vanilla
½ teaspoon ground cinnamon
½ teaspoon turmeric powder
¼ teaspoon freshly grated ginger root
Pinch black pepper
1 tablespoon coconut oil
2 large pitted dates, minced

Preparation
1. Combine all the ingredients in the bowl of a slow cooker.
2. Cook on LOW for 6 hours, until the rice is soft and the milk is absorbed.
3. If is a little dry, you can add more almond milk.

Nutrition facts per serving
Calories 157, total fat 9.9g, carbs 15.5 g, protein 1.6 g, Sodium 0.8 mg, sugar 9.4 g

Berry Cobbler

This is a super simple dessert packed with strawberries and blueberries (fresh or frozen!) and is perfect for summer or winter.

Serves 4 – Preparation time 10 minutes – Cooking time 2 hours

Ingredients

Cobbler Batter

1 cup flour
2 tablespoons sugar
1 teaspoon baking powder
½ teaspoon ground cinnamon
2 bananas, mashed
½ cup coconut or almond milk
2 tablespoons canola oil

Berry Mixture

4 tablespoons flour
1 cup sugar
4 cups mixed berries of choice, fresh or frozen

Preparation
1. Make the batter. In a large bowl, mix the flour, sugar, baking powder, and cinnamon. Stir in the banana, milk, and oil until combined. The batter will be thick.
2. Lightly grease a 4- to 5-quart slow cooker and spread the batter in the bottom.
3. In another large bowl, mix the flour and sugar. Stir in the berries and spread them over the dough in a slow cooker.
4. Cover and cook on HIGH for 2–3 hours (closer to 2 hours for fresh or thawed berries, closer to 3 hours for frozen berries). Serve hot, with a splash of almond milk.

Nutrition facts per serving

Calories 253, total fat 9 g, carbs 42 g, protein 4 g, Sodium 371 mg, sugar 12 g

Mediterranean Stew

Ingredients

1 butternut squash - peeled, seeded, and cubed
2 cups cubed eggplant, with peel
2 cups cubed zucchini
1 (10 ounce) package frozen okra, thawed
1 (8 ounce) can tomato sauce
1 cup chopped onion
1 ripe tomato, chopped
1 carrot, sliced thin
1/2 cup vegetable broth
1/3 cup raisins
1 clove garlic, chopped
1/2 teaspoon ground cumin
1/2 teaspoon ground turmeric
1/4 teaspoon crushed red pepper
1/4 teaspoon ground cinnamon
1/4 teaspoon paprika

Method

1. Combine butternut squash, eggplant, zucchini, okra, tomato sauce, onion, tomato, carrot, raisins and garlic in a slow cooker.
2. Add broth and mix all ingredients together.
3. Adjust seasonings by adding cumin, turmeric, red pepper, cinnamon and paprika.
4. **Cover slow cooker and cook for 8 to 10 hours on a low heat until vegetables are cooked and tender.**

Fennel Soup With White Bean

Ingredients

4 cups Swanson's vegetable broth
1/8 teaspoon ground black pepper
1 small bulb fennel, trimmed and sliced
1 medium onion, chopped
2 cloves garlic, minced
1 (10 ounce) package frozen leaf spinach, thawed
1 (14.5 ounce) can diced tomatoes, undrained
1 (16 ounce) can white kidney beans (cannellini), undrained

Method

1. Place black pepper, fennel, onion and garlic in a slow cooker.
2. Add broth to cooker.
3. Cover and cook on low temperature for 7 hours.
4. **Mix in tomatoes, spinach and beans.**
5. Change heat to high and cook for one hour until vegetables are tender.

"Turks" Eggplants

Ingredients

1/2 cup extra-virgin olive oil

3 small eggplants

Freshly ground black pepper

1 large onion, finely chopped

4 garlic cloves, minced

1 14 1/2- to 15-oz can chopped tomatoes, with their juice

1/4 cup finely chopped fresh flat-leaf parsley

6 8-in round pita breads, quartered and toasted

salt

Method
1. Slice each eggplant lengthwise into halves and slash flesh every ¼" without harming the skin.
2. Pour ¼ cup olive oil into slow cooker and brush cooker with oil.
3. Lay eggplant pieces skin side down and sprinkle with a dash of pepper and salt.
4. **Take a frying pan and heat the balance of the olive oil over medium flame.**
5. Toss onion and garlic and fry for 3 minutes until the onions are transparent in colour.

6. Mix in tomatoes, parsley and adjust salt and pepper; leave for another 5 minutes until liquid is absorbed.
7. Spoon tomato mixture covering about half of eggplant mixture.
8. Cover cooker and cook on high for a little over 2 hours until the eggplant pieces are tender.
9. **Take lid off slow cooker and allow eggplant mixture to rest for about 10 minutes.**
10. Using a spoon, take out eggplant mixture and dish into a serving dish.
11. Pour leftover juice in cooker over the mixture.
12. Serve with toasted pita.

Exotic French Vegetable Soup

Ingredients

2 tablespoons extra-virgin olive oil, plus 1/2 cup

3 leeks (white and tender green parts), halved lengthwise, cleaned, and cut crosswise into 1/2-in half-moons

3 ribs celery, coarsely chopped

3 medium carrots, coarsely chopped

2 teaspoons herbes de Provence

1/2 cup dry white wine, such as Pinot Grigio, Pinot Gris, or Sauvignon Blanc, or dry vermouth

1 14 1/2- to 15-oz can chopped tomatoes, with their juice

8 cups vegetable broth

2 medium zucchini, ends trimmed, and cut into 1/2-in chunks

2 cups fresh shelled peas or frozen peas, defrosted

1 head escarole, cut into 1-in pieces

2 14 1/2- to 15-oz cans small white beans, rinsed and drained

2 cups firmly packed fresh basil leaves

6 garlic cloves, peeled

salt

freshly ground black pepper

Method

1. Pour 2 tbsp olive oil into a pan; temper celery, leeks, carrots and herbes de Provence for a few minutes.
2. Pour in wine and let mixture simmer and cook until liquid reduces a bit.
3. Remove mixture and place in a slow cooker.
4. **Mix in tomatoes, vegetable broth, zucchini, peas, escarole and beans.**
5. Cover cooker and cook for 2 hours on high or for 4 hours on low.
6. Place basil and garlic in a food processor and process on an off until ingredients are broken into pieces.
7. Pour ¼ cup olive oil into the processor.
8. Adjust seasonings by adding salt and pepper as required.

9. **The pistou should hold together but if the consistency is too thick, add a little olive oil.**
10. Remove pistou to a container with a tight lid and pour the balance oil on the surface to prevent basil from staining.
11. Taste the soup and adjust seasonings with salt and pepper.
12. <u>Serve in soup bowls placing 2 tbsp of pistou in the centre of each.</u>
    13. Serve and enjoy.

Three Been Chili

Ingredients

1 can (15 ounces) black beans, rinsed and drained
1 can (15.5 ounces) garbanzo beans, rinsed and drained
1 can (15.5 ounces) kidney beans, rinsed and drained
1 cup dried lentils (8 ounces), sorted and rinsed
1 large vegetarian vegetable cube, crumbled
1 envelope (1.25 ounces) chili seasoning mix
3 cups water
1 can (10 ounces) diced tomatoes and mild green chili, undrained
1 can (15 ounces) tomato sauce

Method

1. Place beans, lentils, vegetable cube, seasoning and water in 3 to 4 quart slow cooker.
2. Cover slow cooker and cook ingredients on low heat for about 10 hours.

3. Insert tomatoes and stir well.
4. **Finally add tomato sauce and increase heat to high.**
5. **Cover cooker and leave for 5-6 minutes until all ingredients are cooked through.**

Crock Pot Mediterranean Stew

Ingredients:
1 butternut squash (peeled, seeded, cubed)
2 cups eggplants (cubed)
2 cups zucchini (cubed)
10 ounces frozen okra (thawed)
8 ounces tomato sauce
1 onion (chopped)
1 carrot (sliced)
1/2 cup vegetable broth
1/3 cup raisins
1 garlic clove (chopped)
1/2 teaspoon cumin
1/2 teaspoon turmeric
1/4 teaspoon crushed red pepper flakes
1/4 teaspoon cinnamon
1/4 teaspoon paprika

Method
1. Insert butternut squash, eggplants, zucchini and okra into a slow cooker. Add onion, tomato sauce, carrot, raisins, and spices.

1. Mix in broth and stir well.
2. **Turn heat to low and allow to cook for 8-9 hours.**

Couscous Mediterranean Stew

Ingredients
1 eggplant, cubed
2 zucchini, cubed
1 butternut squash, cubed
1 onion, chopped
1 tomato, chopped
1 carrot, sliced
1 garlic clove, minced
1/3 cup raisins
1 (14 ounce) can tomato sauce
1/4 cup water
1 teaspoon vegetable stock powder
1/2 teaspoon ground cumin
1/2 teaspoon turmeric
1/4 teaspoon cinnamon
1/4 teaspoon paprika
1/4 teaspoon red pepper flakes

For couscous
3 cups vegetable broth
1/2 teaspoon salt
2 cups couscous

Method

1. Season eggplant with salt, drain in a colander, and set aside for about 20 minutes.
2. Rinse, pat dry, and place in a slow cooker.
3. Add all other ingredients except broth, salt and couscous.
4. **Cook on high for 4 hours.**
5. Combine broth and salt, and bring mixture to a boil.
6. Add couscous, cover the cooker, and reduce heat.
7. Let stand for about 5 minutes and serve hot with stew.

Mediterranean Vegetable Stew

Ingredients
1 medium eggplant, chopped
2 zucchini, chopped
1 red bell peppers or 1 green bell pepper, seeded, diced
1/2 cup onion, chopped
3 large tomatoes, chopped or 1 (14 1/2 ounce) can diced tomatoes
1 tablespoon tomato paste
2 (14 ounce) cans garbanzo beans, drained and rinsed
1 (14 ounce) can water-packed artichoke hearts, drained and quartered
1 1/2 teaspoons dried oregano leaves
fresh ground black pepper

salt
crushed red pepper flakes, to taste

Method
1. Place eggplant, zucchini, bell peppers, onion, tomatoes, beans, artichoke and oregano leaves in a slow cooker.
2. Add tomato paste and adjust seasoning with pepper, salt and pepper flakes.
3. Combine all ingredients and cook on low for 8-9 hours.
4. **Ideal to serve with noodles.**

Delightful Spinach Lentil Soup

Ingredients
1 cup green lentils or 1 cup brown lentils
2 onions, chopped
2 celery ribs, finely chopped
2 carrots, finely chopped
1 potato, peeled and grated
1 clove garlic, minced
1 teaspoon cumin seed
1 teaspoon lemon, zest of
6 cups vegetable broth
1 (10 ounce) package frozen chopped spinach, thawed
2 tablespoons lemon juice

Method
1. Wash lentils with cold water, rinse and drain in a colander.
2. Add washed lentils along with celery, onions, carrots, potato, garlic, cumin seeds and lemon zest into a slow cooker.
3. Pour vegetable broth over other ingredients and combine well.
4. **Cover cooker and cook on low for 9-10 hours or high for 4-6 hours until all ingredients are cooked through.**
5. Finally add spinach and lemon juice; leave for about 20 minutes on a high temperature.

More Delightful Spinach Brown Lentil Soup

Ingredients
1 cup brown lentils
2 onions, chopped
2 celery ribs, chopped
2 carrots, chopped
1 potato, peeled and grated
1 garlic clove, minced
1 teaspoon cumin
1 teaspoon lemon zest
6 cups vegetable broth
salt and pepper to taste

10 ounces frozen spinach
2 tablespoons lemon juice

Method
1. Place all ingredients except spinach and lemon juice in a slow cooker.
2. Cook on low for 8-10 or high for 4-6 hours.
3. Add spinach and lemon juice and stir well.
4. **Cook another 20 minutes on high.**
5. Dish out and serve hot.

Cannellini Bean Soup

Ingredients
1 lb **cannellini beans** (dried, or1 lb dried navy beans)
2 tsps **salt**
8 cups **water**
***2 tbsps** olive oil*
1 **onion** (medium, chopped)
1 **bell pepper** (chopped)
2 **carrots** (chopped)
1 **celery ribs** (chopped)
2 tbsps **garlic** (minced, about 6 cloves)
1 bunch **kale** (fresh)
14 ozs crushed tomatoes
1 tsp dried basil
1 tsp dried rosemary
1/4 tsp red pepper flakes

Method

Wash and drain beans.
Place beans in a slow cooker and add salt and water.
Allow to cook for 8 hours.
Pour oil into a saucepan and keep on medium heat.
Add onion, bell pepper, carrots and celery and cook for 15 minutes until ingredients are tender.
Mix in garlic and let cook for about 4 minutes.
Remove ingredients from saucepan and add to beans in slow cooker
Wash and clean the kale.
Slice the leaves and add to the other ingredients.
Add tomatoes, basil rosemary and red pepper flakes; combine well.
Cook for 20 minutes until kale is cooked tender.

Potato And Bell Pepper Vegetable Stew

Ingredients

2 tbs olive oil
3 shallots **chopped**
1 large carrot **sliced**
2 garlic cloves **minced**
1 pound organic small red potatoes **quartered**
1 organic red bell pepper **seeded and chopped**
9 oz. frozen artichoke hearts
14.5 oz can diced tomatoes
1 1/2 cups cooked chickpeas
1/3 cup dry white wine

1 1/2 cups vegetable stock
1 tsp fresh thyme leaves **minced or 1/4 tsp dried**
1 tsp fresh oregano leaves **minced or 1/4 tsp dried**
1 large bay leaf
salt and pepper

Method
1. Pour oil into slow cooker and heat a bit.
2. Add shallots, carrots, and garlic; sauté until ingredients are soft.
3. Add balance of ingredients and combine well.
4. **Cover and cook for 6-8 hours on low until all ingredients are cooked through.**

Yummy Artichoke Pasta

Ingredients
nonstick cooking spray
3 x 14 1/2 ounce cans diced tomatoes with basil, oregano, and garlic
2 x 14 ounce cans artichoke hearts, drained and quartered
6 cloves garlic**, minced**
½ cup coconut cream
12 ounces dried linguine, fettuccini, or other favorite pasta
sliced pimiento-stuffed green olives and/or sliced pitted ripe olives (optional)
crumbled soy cheese

Method
1. Cook pasta, drain and set aside.
2. Coat inside of slow cooker with cooking spray.
3. Drain 2 cans of diced tomatoes and add to slow cooker.
4. **Mix in other undrained can of tomatoes, artichokes, and garlic.**
5. Cover and cook for 6-8 hours on low heat for 3-4 hours.
6. Mix in coconut cream and combine well, allowing to stand for a few minutes.
7. Serve mixture over cooked pasta and serve with olives and soy cheese.

The White Man Spread

Ingredients
2 x 15 ounce cans Great Northern or cannellini (white kidney) beans, rinsed and drained
½ cup vegetable broth
1 tablespoon olive oil
3 cloves garlic**, minced**
1 teaspoon snipped *fresh marjoram*
½ teaspoon snipped *fresh rosemary*
1/8 teaspoon ground black pepper
 olive oil
 fresh marjoram leaves and rosemary (optional)
 assorted crackers

Method

1. Place beans, broth, olive oil, garlic, ½ tsp marjoram, ½ tsp rosemary and pepper in a slow cooker.
2. Cover and cook for 3-4 hours on low heat.
3. Dish out and squash mixture using potato masher.
4. **Place in serving bowls with garmosj, fresh marjoram, and rosemary leaves on top.**
5. Serve with crackers.

Wintery Soup With Squash And Chickpea

Ingredients

2 medium onions, peeled and chopped
2 pounds butternut, acorn, or other winter squash, peeled and cut into chunks
1 cup peeled, seeded and chopped fresh tomatoes, or canned tomatoes
2 cups cooked or canned chickpeas, drained
2 cups vegetable broth or water
3 cups water
Salt and freshly ground pepper
2 tablespoons vegan margarine
chopped cilantro, mint, or Italian parsley

Method

1. Insert onions, squash, tomatoes and chick peas into slow cooker.
2. Add broth along with 1 tsp of salt and pepper and combine well.

3. Cover and cook for 4 hours on high or for 8 hours on low until ingredients are cooked.
4. **Place vegetables and chickpeas in a blender and process for a few minutes.**
5. Mix in the vegan margarine and adjust seasonings.
6. Sprinkle with herbs and serve hot.

The Amazing Minestrone Casserole

Ingredients

3 medium carrots, sliced (1 1/2 cups)
1 medium onion, chopped (1/2 cup)
1 cup water
2 teaspoons sugar
1 teaspoon Italian seasoning
½ teaspoon salt
¼ teaspoon pepper
1 can (28 ounces) diced tomatoes, not drained
1 can (15 oz) Progresso garbanzo beans, rinsed and drained
1 can (6 ounces) Italian-style tomato paste
2 cloves garlic, finely chopped
1 ½ cups Green Giant Steamers frozen cut green beans (from 12 oz bag), thawed
1 cup uncooked elbow macaroni (3 1/2 ounces)

Method
1. Place all ingredients except green beans, macaroni into a slow cooker.
2. Cover and allow to cook on low for 6-8 hours.

3. Mix in green beans and macaroni.
4. **Increase heat to high, cover and cook for 20 minutes until ingredients are tender.**
5. **Serve hot.**

Bulgur And Lentils

Ingredients

1 cup uncooked bulgur or cracked wheat
½ cup dried lentils, sorted, rinsed
1 teaspoon ground cumin
¼ teaspoon salt
3 cloves garlic, finely chopped
1 can (15.25 oz) whole kernel corn, drained
2 cans (14 oz each) vegetable broth
2 medium tomatoes, chopped (1 1/2 cups)
½ cup drained pitted kalamata olives

Method

1. Place all ingredients except tomatoes and olives into a slow cooker.
2. Cover and cook on low for 3-4 hours until lentils are cooked and tender.
3. Mix in tomatoes, olives and increase heat to high.
4. **Cover and cook for 15-20 minutes.**
5. Remove from cooker and serve hot.

Greek-Style Veggies

Ingredients

1 medium zucchini, cut into 1/2-inch slices (4 cups)
1 medium eggplant, peeled and cut into 1/2-inch cubes (4 cups)
1 medium red bell pepper, cut into strips
1 medium onion, chopped (1/2 cup)
3 package (8 ounces) whole mushrooms, cut into fourths
1 cloves garlic, finely chopped
1 can (28 ounces) tomato puree, undrained
1 can (2 1/4 ounces) sliced ripe olives, drained
2 teaspoons salt
2 teaspoons dried basil leaves
½ teaspoon dried thyme leaves
¼ teaspoon pepper

Method

1. Place all ingredients in a slow cooker and combine well.
2. Cover and cook on low for 7-8 hours until ingredients are tender.
3. Remove from cooker and serve hot.

Mr. Three Vegetarian Chili

Ingredients

2 cans (14 oz each) vegetable broth
1 cup chopped onion (1 large)
¼ cup chopped seeded jalapeño chiles
2 teaspoons chili powder

2 teaspoons ground cumin
2 teaspoons Worcestershire sauce
½ teaspoon salt
2 cloves garlic, finely chopped
2 cans (15 oz each) Progresso black beans, drained, rinsed
2 cans (14.5 oz each) Muir Glen organic diced tomatoes, not drained
1 can (15 to 16 oz) pinto beans, drained, rinsed
1 can (15 oz) Progresso red kidney beans, drained, rinsed
½ cup vegan sour cream
½ cup shredded soy cheese (2 oz)
1/4 cup chopped fresh cilantro

Method
1. Use a cooking spray in the slow cooker.
2. Place all ingredients except vegan sour cream, soy cheese, and cilantro in cooker.
3. Combine ingredients.
4. **Cover and cook on low for 8 hours.**
5. Remove from cooker and serve hot.
6. Use a little of the sour cream, soy cheese, and cilantro to top each serving.

The Brave Vegan Chili

Ingredients
1 (12 ounce) package vegetarian burger crumbles
3 (15.25 ounce) cans kidney beans

1 large red onion, chopped
4 stalks celery, diced
2 red bell peppers, chopped
4 bay leaves
2 tablespoons hot chili powder
3 tablespoons molasses
1 cube vegetable bouillon
1 tablespoon chopped fresh cilantro
1 teaspoon hot pepper sauce
salt and pepper to taste
1 cup water
3 tablespoons all-purpose flour
1 cup hot water

Method
1. Place vegetarian crumbles, onion, kidney beans, celery, bell peppers, bay leaves, molasses, bouillon, cilantro, spices and sauce in a slow cooker.
2. Add water, adjust seasonings with salt and pepper, and cook for 3 hours on high heat.
3. Mix flour with 1 cup hot water and once dissolved add to rest of ingredients in slow cooker
4. **Leave for one more hour until all ingredients are cooked through.**
5. Serve hot.

Delicious Mediterranean Tomato Sauce

Ingredients
10 plum tomatoes - peeled, seeded and crushed

1/2 small onion, chopped
1 teaspoon minced garlic
1/4 cup olive oil
1 teaspoon dried oregano
1 teaspoon dried basil
1 teaspoon ground cayenne pepper
1 teaspoon salt
1 teaspoon ground black pepper
1 pinch cinnamon

Method
- In a slow cooker, place tomatoes, onion, garlic and olive oil.
- Add basil, oregano, pepper, salt, black pepper and cinnamon and combine well.
- Cover and cook for 10-15 hours on low heat.

Spiced Apple Sauce

Ingredients
8 apples - peeled, cored, and thinly sliced
1/2 cup water
3/4 cup packed brown sugar
1/2 teaspoon pumpkin pie spice

Method
1. In a slow cooker, place the apples and water.
2. Cook for 6-8 hours on low heat.
3. Mix in sugar and spice.

4. **Stir well and keep on heat for another ½ hour.**

Garbanzo Chili

Ingredients

1 (28 ounce) can whole peeled tomatoes with juice
1 (15 ounce) can garbanzo beans, drained
2 zucchini, thinly sliced
1 onion, chopped
2 carrots, sliced
2 stalks celery, sliced
1 red bell pepper, chopped
1 green bell pepper, chopped
1/3 cup chili powder
1 (4 ounce) can chopped green chili peppers
2 cloves garlic, minced
1 tablespoon dried oregano
2 teaspoons ground cumin
1 teaspoon salt

Method
1. Place beans, zucchini, onion, carrots, celery, red pepper, green pepper, chili powder, chili peppers, garlic, oregano, cumin and salt in a slow cooker.
2. Add tomatoes with juice and combine well.
3. Cover and cook for 6-8 hours on low heat.
4. **Dish out when all ingredients are cooked; serve hot.**

The Spinach Lover's Marinara Sauce

Ingredients

1/4 cup olive oil
1 onion, chopped
5 cloves garlic, minced
1/3 cup grated carrot
1 (10 ounce) package frozen chopped spinach, thawed and drained
2 2/3 (6 ounce) cans tomato paste
1 (4.5 ounce) can sliced mushrooms, drained
2 tablespoons salt
2 tablespoons dried oregano
2 tablespoons dried basil
2 1/2 tablespoons crushed red pepper
2 bay leaves
1 (28 ounce) can peeled and crushed tomatoes, with liquid

Method

1. Place spinach in a slow cooker.
2. Add olive oil, onion, garlic, carrot, tomato paste, mushrooms, basil, oregano, red pepper, bay leaves, and tomatoes, salt and mix well.
3. Cover and cook for 4 hours on high heat.
4. **Combine ingredients and reduce heat to low.**
5. Cook for 1-2 hours until ingredients are cooked.

Delicious Root Vegetable Tagine

Ingredients
1 pound parsnips, peeled and diced
1 pound turnips, peeled and diced
2 medium onions, chopped
1 pound carrots, peeled and diced
6 dried apricots, chopped
4 pitted prunes, chopped
1 teaspoon ground turmeric
1 teaspoon ground cumin
1/2 teaspoon ground ginger
1/2 teaspoon ground cinnamon
1/4 teaspoon ground cayenne pepper
1 tablespoon dried parsley
1 tablespoon dried cilantro
1 (14 ounce) can vegetable broth

Method
1. Place parsnips, turnips, onions, carrots, apricots and prunes in the slow cooker.
2. Pour in vegetable broth over ingredients.
3. Add turmeric, cumin, ginger, cinnamon, cayenne pepper, parsley and cilantro and mix well
4. **Cover and cook on low for 8-9 hours.**

Grandma's Vegetarian Chili

Ingredients
1 (19 ounce) can black bean soup

1 (15 ounce) can kidney beans, rinsed and drained
1 (15 ounce) can garbanzo beans, rinsed and drained
1 (16 ounce) can vegetarian baked beans
1 (14.5 ounce) can chopped tomatoes in puree
1 (15 ounce) can whole kernel corn, drained
1 onion, chopped
1 green bell pepper, chopped
2 stalks celery, chopped
2 cloves garlic, chopped
1 tablespoon chili powder, or to taste
1 tablespoon dried parsley
1 tablespoon dried oregano
1 tablespoon dried basil

Method
1. Pour black bean soup into a slow cooker.
2. Toss kidney beans, garbanzo beans, baked beans, oregano and basil into the soup.
3. Adjust seasoning with garlic, chili powder, parsley, oregano and basil.
4. **Cover and cook on high for 2 hours.**

Black Beans And Rice

Ingredients
1 lb dried black beans (2 cups), sorted, rinsed
1 large onion, chopped (1 cup)
1 large bell pepper, chopped (1 1/2 cups)
5 cloves garlic, finely chopped
2 dried bay leaves

1 can (14.5 oz) Muir Glen organic diced tomatoes, undrained
5 cups water
2 tablespoons olive or vegetable oil
4 teaspoons ground cumin
2 teaspoons finely chopped jalapeño chilies
1 teaspoon salt
3 cups hot cooked rice

Method
1. Place black beans, onion, bell pepper, garlic, bay leaves, tomatoes, oil, cumin, chili and salt in a slow cooker.
2. Add water and mix well.
3. Cover cooker and cook for 6-8 hours on high.
4. **Dish out beans (ensure to remove bay leaves).**
5. Serve with rice.